The Hospice Way of Death

The Hospice Way of Death

Paul M. DuBois, PhD

Tennessee State University
Nashville, Tennessee

HUMAN SCIENCES PRESS

72 Fifth Avenue   3 Henrietta Street
NEW YORK, NY 10011 ● LONDON, WC2E 8LU

Printed in the United States of America
0 1 2 3 4 5 6 7 8 9

Library of Congress Cataloging in Publication Data

DuBois, Paul M
   The hospice way of death.

   Bibliography: p.
   Includes index.
   1. Terminal care. 2. Terminal care facilities.
3. Terminal care—United States. I. Title.
R726.8.D85   616   LC 79–12326
ISBN 0-87705-415-0

To Joan,
who died with dignity and love.

Acknowledgements

While many people contributed to this book, special thanks must go to:

Mrs. Nancy DuBois

Dr. Frederick T. Bent

Dr. Tom E. Davis

Dr. Michael Latham

Ms. Claire Ravizza

Ms. Constance Adler

Contents

1. Introduction: What Is a Hospice?   11
2. The Causes of Death   21
3. The Quality of Dying in America   37
4. Components of Hospice Care   60
5. Case Study I: St. Christopher's Hospice   69
6. Case Study II: Hospice, Inc.   85
7. Case Study III: Strong Memorial
   Hospital—A Failure to Start
   a Hospice   111
8. The Hospice Movement   133
9. The Federal Response   139
   Notes   169
   Bibliography   187
   Index   209

1

Introduction:

What Is a Hospice?

Hospices, first and foremost, comprise a movement. They are urged upon the American public by people living in 80 cities across the nation. These advocates want to establish special programs for dying people who need help to die peacefully at home, and people who wish to be removed to a separate facility during their last days. Regardless of where death occurs, hospice care is intended to make the last weeks and months of our lives easy to bear and free from pain and fear. Because it boasts such a lofty purpose, the movement deserves study and public discussion.

This book is designed to encourage that discussion by providing a comprehensive examination of the hospice movement while it is still in a developmental stage. Planners, physicians, and other professionals concerned with health care in the United States, as well as lay people who pay for that care, should be aware of attempts to impose new medical institutions upon a system that already delivers highly specialized, sophisticated, and very expensive care.

The term "hospice" as defined by professional planners of the hospice movement means:[1]

> A program which provides palliative and supportive care for terminally ill patients and their families, either directly or on a consulting basis with the patient's physician or another community agency such as a visiting nurse association. Originally a medieval name for a way station for pilgrims and travelers where they could be replenished, refreshed, and cared for; used here for an organized program of care for people going through life's last station. The whole family is considered the unit of care and care extends through the mourning process. Emphasis is placed on symptom control and preparation for and support before and after death, full scope health services being provided by an organized interdisciplinary team available on a twenty-four-hours-a-day, seven-days-a-week basis. Hospices originated in England (where there are about 25) and are now appearing in the United States. As one example of their human and cost-saving effects, 61 percent of one hospice's patients die at home (compared with the two percent of all American deaths which occur at home).

Some of the goals of hospice care implied in this definition are not new to those people concerned with the quality of health care. Long before the birth of Christ, Plato in his *Republic* recommended family involvement and a sympathetic approach towards people in extreme personal distress. The Belgian Gheel community has provided foster home care since the Middle Ages. And a few hospices have been located throughout Europe, serving as homes for dying people, for a century. By and large, however, the majority of nonwealthy families in Western society during the past several centuries have had to rely upon very meager resources during the stages of dying. Indeed, historians note that the principal publicly financed institutions coming in contact with dying people have been the work-houses, lunatic asylums, houses of correction, and prisons that combine to make for a sordid history of gross insensitivity to the needs of people during the last stage of life.[2]

Small wonder, then, that some of the leading figures in the modern hospice movement have searched into the fear-ridden past to select a comforting name for their objectives. Edward Dobihal, Chairperson of the Board of Directors of Hospice, Inc. describes the use of the word hospice among his planning staff in New Haven:[3]

> Hospice means a community of people with a common goal—to care for travelers on the way. We chose the name because it is most appropriate for the person resting and finding refreshment and renewal in concluding the journey of life. We also chose the name because of its international usage since several of our group have visited and studied at St. Christopher's Hospice, a terminal care facility in London, learning much that has helped us in our philosophy and planning.

> The planning group has stated their philosophy in part as follows: "The professional and scientific knowledge of nursing and medicine combined with this reverence for life and its spirit, serve to help the staff understand the experiences of the patient and his family to relieve their distress. We find that this type of care increases the capacity of the patient and his family to live through this period with meaning and dignity."

This book will describe the burgeoning hospice movement and explore a number of issues regarding how hospices fit into existing community mental health and intensive care systems. It will examine the considerable gap between the needs of a widespread local movement organized to deliver a new type of health care and the federal government's undeveloped responses that lack coordination, rational planning, and an understanding of the consequences of federal policy for the quality of dying in this country. The author will try to determine whether hospices are a rational, cost-efficient addition to community health support systems as presently organized in the United States.

That hospices represent an important response to current needs is suggested by the statements of such researchers as Judith Kohn:[4]

> The dying don't press their needs. Their families don't cry out much either. And, for a variety of reasons ranging from ignorance to insensitivity, most health care providers are doing little or nothing to improve the lot of terminally ill patients in hospitals and elsewhere. Indeed, it is becoming increasingly clear that in most parts of the United States and Canada, these patients do not receive appropriate services. Thus, inadequate care of the dying represents a significant gap in our health care system.
>
> The void exists partly because acute care hospitals are ill-suited to meet the physical and emotional needs of the dying, who must watch their own deterioration and the slow approach of death over a period of weeks or months. Such institutions are geared instead to cure patients and send them home as quickly as possible and to give efficient rather than individually optimized care.
>
> Hospice goals differ markedly from those of acute care facilities that focus on investigation, diagnosis and cure. In contrast to traditional medical goals, a major aim of a hospice program is palliation of symptoms so that patients can live out their lives as comfortably and meaningfully as possible.

Kohn points out that hospice care goes far beyond palliation, but the supplementary and alternative nature of hospices, as places to receive a specialized therapy that traditional institutions cannot provide, is what interests us. Hospital design consultant John Thompson states:[5]

> The old idea of one hospital to satisfy all needs is a thing of the past. . . . We need a *series* of institutions. We'll always need

some health-care factories for efficient, short-term, intensive-care stays, but we'll need others where humanity won't have to overcome the technical apparatus.

In the terminal situation, the family is as necessary as any other form of care. But we exclude families from intensive-care units. The hospice represents one type of facility where family interaction is possible.

The two best ways to determine the significance (or insignificance) of hospices as an element in a rational community health support system are from the perspectives of both the individual patient and the community mental health planner. Research on the needs of dying patients in various settings will be reviewed. On the basis of that assessment, what portion of the dying population most needs hospices can be determined, and we can form some conclusions about whether the components of hospice care actually meet the needs of dying people.

Constance Holder notes that,[6]

Of the 700,000 people diagnosed as having cancer each year, two out of three die of their malignancies. For these people dying can be a slow, painful, and very lonely business ... Despite the growing concern about death and dying in this country, there is not much public understanding of the needs of dying people—the needs for comfort both physical and mental, for others to see them as individuals rather than as hosts of their diseases, for someone to breach the loneliness and help them come to terms with the end.

Meeting or not meeting the needs of individual dying patients provides an important perspective from which to evaluate the usefulness of hospices. The second perspective, that of the community health care planner, questions whether hospices have a place within the community's "support system." Hospice planners have addressed this issue with some anxiety:[7]

liaison with community agencies has been a touchy problem in terms of details. It is important to emphasize to them that the Hospice is there to back up their services, not to duplicate them. The Visiting Nurses and similar organizations should not be made to feel threatened.

Hospice, Inc., in New Haven, Connecticut makes a case for hospices by describing the inadequacies of four well-developed elements of the existing community support system:[8]

Hospitals

Hospitals are, practically and philosophically, oriented to the cure of disease. This immediate urgency guides the hospital's efforts. The staff and most of the other resources are devoted to helping the patient recover from disease.

When disease cannot be cured, the hospital has few resources to help the patient live as fully and completely as possible; nor can it give the patient's family the skilled care and support they need to understand and cope with the effects of this continuing illness.

Nursing and Convalescent Homes

Most nursing and convalescent homes are not equipped to give additional priority attention to the physical and emotional needs of the terminally ill, much less to their families. These institutions are designed primarily to provide long term care for the elderly and to conclude a recuperative period of rehabilitative program for patients.

Care for the elderly is essential, but for the 50% of those patients suffering from cancer who are under sixty-five years of age, the nursing home environment is inappropriate . . .

For the terminally ill, cure is an unrealistic goal, and many rehabilitation programs refuse admission to those with a short prognosis.

The terminally ill need very specialized and concentrated medical and nursing services, as well as varied support services for psychological, social, and spiritual stress. Family members also benefit from such support.

Health Care Professionals

Until very recently, most of the professionals' training and viewpoint have been oriented to the treatment of disease and the preservation of life.

When professionals come face-to-face with the reality of a dying patient, his needs, life style, and specific requests, they must often struggle with the biases of past training, the orientation of health care agencies, and their concern for the patient and for the family.

Health care professionals, like many people, have difficulty coming to terms with the inevitability of dying.

Counseling

The care of the terminally ill is incomplete without counseling—both to the patient and the family. Often the focus has been only on the patient. But as noted authority Dr. Elizabeth Kubler-Ross points out, the acceptance of death is often more difficult for the patient's family than it is for the patient himself. Help must be available for both.

Clergy have long filled the role of friend of the family, but counseling other than spiritual—financial, practical, emotional—is often unavailable, especially on an ongoing basis. Death involves more than prayers and tears—it is a web of insurance policies, bills, attorneys, physicians, guilt, loss of income and funeral preparations. To help the patient/family cope with the reality of impending death, supportive relationships during the illness are necessary. To ease the pain of separation and grief and to assist in creating a new life for the family, this care must continue during their time of bereavement.

Do these statements accurately depict the inadequacy of present health care institutions to meet the needs of the dying? Is there a "health care gap" large enough to justify the years of planning and millions of dollars now being allocated to hospice development throughout the United States? These are two of the issues that will be addressed in subsequent chapters of this book.

Another important aspect of hospices concerns the care given to *the families* of the dying. Joan Craven and Florence Wald state:[9]

> Grieving begins before death occurs and continues after death. Patient, family, friends, and those who give care all experience the sorrow to some degree; they all need comfort. The bereaved are more vulnerable to physical and psychological disease; care for the survivors, therefore, is as legitimate a concern of health professionals as preventive medicine. It begins while caring for the patient and is needed until the survivors can cope for themselves, or until other resources such as mental health services, family physician, extended family, or minister are found to provide the help still needed. The grieving processes of separation are far better understood than they were 10 years ago; as a result, we are better able to help.

The interesting question of whether there is a benefit from hospice care in terms of preventive medicine for the survivors has not been answered in the literature. No experimental and control groups have been studied, but the needs of families experiencing the dying process have been researched, and the likelihood that hospice care will meet those needs can be reasonably analyzed.

Besides looking at individual needs, this book will also examine the gap between the needs of a widespread local movement organized to deliver a new type of health care and the federal government's undeveloped responses. It appears likely that the federal government, as represented by the Department of Health, Education and Welfare and the National Institute of Health, is not presently organized to devise and implement coordinated, comprehensive policies regarding the development of hospices. Instead, the federal government lacks understanding of the impact of federal policy making on the quality of dying in this country as well as structures capable of responding rationally to a growing movement that expects to deliver a new type of health care. What federal agencies presently respond to the pressures to develop hospices? How do they respond? Can we make any recommendations to improve the response? Can a case be made to take the subject of the quality of death "out of the closet" and into the public discourse by establishing governmental agencies to formulate public policy and even to draft relevant legislation?

The subject of hospices is an important, recent example of how the death process is publicly ignored in the United States. Death and dying are only indirectly included in American policy debates regarding health care delivery. Lay and many professional people persist in a perception of death as essentially a personal and private matter, that is, a crisis with which each individual must cope using the very limited resources available in modern society.

It is our concept—some say our fear—of death that constitutes one reason why hospices are subtly opposed in our country. In addition, we are content to leave the management of death to hospital staff, without ever examining whether the hospital setting is the appropriate place for people who have no chance of cure, no matter how heroic the treatment. Hospices are threatening to people who know little of the demographics and quality of dying in America. Hospices represent an innovation, something with which we are not familiar. Because they are not part of the public health program so widely accepted in our country, there is little community support for them.

The literature on death and dying available to professionals also fails to examine the impact of public programs and policies that influence the quality of dying in America and deals almost exclusively with medical care of the dying and the process of mourning. The psychological, medical, and public health literature frequently notes the impact of health care policies on the medical characteristics of dying in America since the turn of the century. Epidemics no longer take a great toll of human lives. Morbidity and mortality rates in infancy and early childhood have been drastically reduced. Many diseases have been conquered in the past several decades, and the development of antibiotics and chemotherapies means that many infectious diseases no longer produce widespread fatalities. A high proportion of our population die from malignancies and chronic diseases, and the number of older people, often with decreased capacities, continues to rise. Indeed, the number of living people over the age of 65 increase at the rate of 1,000 per day. There were 365,000 more senior citizens in the United States in any recent year than there were the previous year. The professional literature indicates some concern with such macro issues as technology transformation and alternative technologies in the professional "mix" of services, demographic changes, and broad, socially-induced changes in family structures, while the popular media, as we all know, have treated the subject of euthanasia superficially.

The impact of these developments on public policy making in America and the impact of public policies and public administration on the quality of dying in this country have not been thoroughly studied in a way that might affect both the substance of the policy process and the manner in which it is carried out. This book, then, provides a description of the hospice movement and an analysis of the potential impact of hospices upon the quality of dying in this country.

2

The Causes of Death

Quite obviously, we all will die. But many of us live longer than others, and the causes of death have changed dramatically during the last several decades. The answer to the question "Who will die this year?" has been changing in America for some time. Mortality and morbidity data can offer a description of just which Americans die and when.

The general trends in mortality characteristics in America are known for most of its history. The average lifetime in the United States by the mid-19th century was about 40 years.[1] The discovery of the bacterial origin of disease during the half century before 1900 meant that outbreaks of yellow fever, cholera, and smallpox were gradually brought under control. Since 1900, mortality rates have been high in the first year of life, falling rapidly to a low point near age 10, slowly rising again to about age 45, and then rising rapidly after that.[2] This trend holds over sex and race during the first six decades of this century as evident in Table 1.[3]

Table 1
Mortality Rates per 1,000 and Expectation of Life at Specified Ages, by Sex and Race in the United States from 1900 to 1964

Calendar Period	Mortality Rate per 1,000					Expectation of Life, Years				
	Age 0	Age 10	Age 20	Age 45	Age 65	Age 0	Age 10	Age 20	Age 45	Age 65
White Males										
1900–02*	133.5	2.7	5.9	12.6	41.7	48.2	50.6	42.2	24.2	11.5
1909–11*	123.3	2.4	4.9	12.6	43.8	50.2	51.3	42.7	23.9	11.3
1919–21†	80.3	2.1	4.3	9.3	35.0	56.3	54.2	45.6	26.0	12.2
1929–31	62.3	1.5	3.2	9.3	38.7	59.1	55.0	46.0	25.3	11.8
1939–41	48.1	1.0	2.1	7.7	36.9	62.8	57.0	47.8	25.9	12.1
1949–51	30.7	0.6	1.6	6.4	34.5	66.3	59.0	49.5	26.9	12.8
1959–61	25.9	0.4	1.6	5.6	33.9	67.6	59.8	50.3	27.3	13.0
1964	24.5	0.3	1.6	5.5	34.4	67.7	59.8	50.2	27.4	13.0
White Females										
1900–02*	110.6	2.5	5.5	10.6	36.4	51.1	52.2	43.8	25.5	12.2
1901–11	102.3	2.1	4.9	9.9	37.9	53.6	53.6	44.9	25.5	12.0
1919–21†	63.9	1.8	4.3	8.1	31.7	58.5	55.2	46.5	27.0	12.8
1929–31	49.6	1.1	2.8	7.0	31.3	62.7	57.7	48.5	27.4	12.8
1939–41	37.9	0.7	1.5	5.2	26.4	67.3	60.9	51.4	28.9	13.6
1949–51	23.6	0.4	0.7	3.7	20.6	72.0	64.3	54.6	31.1	15.0
1959–61	19.6	0.3	0.6	3.0	17.4	74.2	66.1	56.3	32.5	15.9
1964	18.6	0.3	0.6	3.0	16.9	74.6	66.4	56.6	32.9	16.3
Nonwhite Males‡										
1919–21†	105.0	2.7	10.9	17.1	38.9	47.1	46.0	38.4	23.6	12.1
1929–31	87.3	2.1	8.6	22.4	50.7	47.6	44.3	36.0	20.6	10.9
1939–41	82.3	1.4	5.4	18.6	46.9	52.3	48.3	39.5	21.9	12.2
1949–51	50.9	0.8	3.1	12.9	45.8	58.9	53.0	43.7	23.6	12.8
1959–61	47.0	0.6	2.4	10.4	43.7	61.5	55.2	45.8	24.9	12.8
1964	45.7	0.5	2.4	11.1	49.6	61.1	54.7	45.3	24.7	12.8
Nonwhite Females‡										
1919–21†	87.5	2.9	11.6	18.7	43.4	46.9	44.5	37.2	22.6	12.4
1929–31	72.0	1.6	8.8	20.2	49.4	49.5	45.3	37.2	21.4	12.2
1939–41	65.8	1.0	5.3	16.0	40.9	55.6	50.8	42.0	23.9	13.9
1949–51	40.9	0.6	2.3	11.3	37.0	62.7	56.2	46.8	26.1	14.5
1959–61	38.3	0.4	1.2	7.7	30.7	66.5	59.7	50.1	28.1	15.1
1964	36.8	0.4	1.1	7.4	35.5	67.2	60.3	50.6	28.7	15.6

* Original death registration states.
† Death registration states of 1920.
‡ Blacks only before 1949.
Source: Bureau of the Census and the National Center for Health Statistics.

There have been striking gains in the expectation of life. The expected life span increased for white males by 19.5 years between 1900 and 1964. Women have enjoyed a more rapid reduction in death rates than males, and the gain in expected life span for white females from 1900 to 1964 was 23.5 years. Black people suffer from significantly higher mortality rates than whites, particularly in infancy and among women. The mortality statistics have been improving for blacks more rapidly than for whites, but the differences remain substantial.

Some other trends not shown in Table 1 can be mentioned here.[4] Mortality for married people is lower than that for unmarried people at each age level (perhaps because marriage is a selective process or because married people may receive better care when sick). Mortality declines, too, as one moves up the socioeconomic ladder as defined by jobs. Environmental influences as well as occupational hazards may cause earlier deaths among laborers than among professional people. Mortality rates in infancy are also highest in the Mountain States and lowest in New England and the mid-Atlantic States. Mortality also differs by age and sex over the states, with farming populations generally doing better than foreign-born and industrial populations.

As noted earlier, the greatest reductions in mortality have been brought about by better nutrition and the control of infectious diseases. Table 2 compares leading causes of death in 1900 and 1964.[5] Cardiovascular-renal conditions and cancer are now the leading causes of death. At the turn of the century they were far less significant.

The significant changes in mortality by selected causes during roughly the first six decades of this century are usually attributed to the rising standard of living including nutritional status, the increased availability of medical services, the development of health facilities, the public health movement which had its greatest impact on sanitary and preventive measures such as innoculations,

Table 2
The Ten Leading Causes of
Death in the United States, 1900 and 1964

Rank	Cause of Death	Death Rate per 100,000 Population	Percent of Deaths from All Causes
	1900		
1.	Pneumonia and influenza	202	11.8
2.	Tuberculosis	194	11.3
3.	Diarrhea and enteritis	143	8.3
4.	Diseases of the heart	137	8.0
5.	Cerebral hemorrhage	107	6.2
6.	Nephritis	89	5.2
7.	Accidents	72	4.2
8.	Cancer	64	3.7
9.	Diphtheria	40	2.3
10.	Meningitis	34	2.0
	1964		
1.	Diseases of the heart	366	38.9
2.	Cancer and other malignancies	151	16.1
3.	Cerebral hemorrhage	104	11.0
4.	Accidents	54	5.8
5.	Certain diseases of early infancy	32	3.4
6.	Pneumonia and influenza (except of newborn)	31	3.3
7.	General arteriosclerosis	19	2.1
8.	Diabetes mellitus	17	1.8
9.	Other diseases of circulatory system	14	1.4
10.	Other bronchopulmonic diseases	12	1.3

Source: National Center for Health Statistics.

and major advances in chemotherapy and pharmacology. All of these factors have resulted in a declining problem of orphanhood and a growing problem of widowhood. Indeed, perhaps the most serious social problems of the dying occur among women who are longer members of households because their husbands have died, and among families of all ages in which a parent (often the breadwinner) is dying of one of our modern diseases such as cancer. Hospice care may be particularly useful to people in both groups.

Having briefly looked at mortality trends for the first half of the century, it may be instructive to examine more closely (1) the status of older Americans, who are increasing as a proportion of our population; (2) mortality trends for the two decades immediately preceding the 1970s, so that we can move from the perspective of a full half century to that of very recent history; and (3) statistics on deaths caused by cancer, since the proportion of cancer patients in the dying population has greatly increased in recent decades and they often are considered prime candidates for hospice care.

The number of Americans age 65 and over has increased significantly over the years, as indicated in Table 3.[6] As might be expected, the proportion of the aged at the extreme edge of life is also rising, so that while 30 percent were over the age of 75 in 1940, 38 percent were in this range in 1975. Furthermore, females are gaining more rapidly than males in the upper age brackets. To be suddenly left alone after the death of a spouse presents many social and economic problems, especially for older people and particularly for those living at home under their own care. Economic consequences of death may fall most severely on surviving women.

The increasing proportion of older Americans within the general population, as well as the proportion of the very aged (over 75) among the older population itself, suggest that Americans who are dying increasingly require

Table 3

Shifts in the Age and Sex Distribution of the Population of the
United States Since 1920 with Projection to 1980

Year	Population, Thousands		Percent of Total at Ages		Ratio: Females per 100 Males			
	All Ages	Ages 65 and Over	65 and Over	75 and Over	All Ages	Under Age 65	Ages 65–74	Ages 75 and Over
1920	105,711	4,933	4.7	1.4	96.1	96.0	93.9	110.9
1930	122,775	6,634	5.4	1.6	97.6	97.5	95.9	108.8
1940	131,820	8,969	6.8	2.9	99.1	98.7	101.3	113.2
1950	151,132	12,194	8.1	2.6	100.8	99.9	107.3	121.1
1959	177,103	15,380	8.7	3.0	102.1	100.4	114.9	132.8
1965	193,643	17,638	9.1	3.3	102.6	100.4	121.7	139.5
1970	208,199	19,549	9.4	3.5	102.9	100.3	125.3	146.5
1975	225,552	21,872	9.7	3.7	103.0	100.0	127.1	153.0
1980	245,409	24,526	10.0	3.8	102.9	99.5	128.9	157.4

Source: Speigelman, M. *Ensuring medical care for the aged*, p. 5.[7]

the terminal care associated with the practices of gerontology rather than heroic life-preserving measures often
found in hospitals. The very high proportion of these older
Americans who live in families (75 percent of males and
66 percent of females over age 75) suggests that there may
be important financial, social, and psychological reasons
why terminal care provided to the aged should be family
based, making use of outpatient services. There seems to
be no reason to disrupt the life-styles of this large proportion of dying Americans.

We can rank the most recent leading causes of death in
the general American population by order of incidence.[8]
For the two decades from 1950 to 1969, cancer, diabetes,
emphysema, cirrhosis of the liver, suicide, and homicide
rates have all been increasing.[9]

Those causes of death requiring terminal care of the
type delivered by hospices would not, of course, include
accidents, suicides, or homicides. When all other causes of

Table 4
Mortality for Leading Causes of Death: United States, 1973

Rank	Cause of Death	Number of Deaths	Death Rate per 100,000 Population	Percent of Total Deaths
	All Causes	1,973,003	940.2	100.0
1.	Diseases of heart	757,075	360.8	38.4
2.	Cancer	351,055	167.3	17.8
3.	Stroke	214,313	102.1	10.9
4.	Accidents	115,821	55.2	5.9
5.	Influenza and pneumonia	62,559	29.8	3.2
6.	Diabetes Mellitus	38,208	18.2	1.9
7.	Cirrhosis of liver	33,350	15.9	1.7
8.	Arteriosclerosis	32,617	15.5	1.7
9.	Certain diseases of infancy	30,503	14.5	1.5
10.	Suicide	25,118	12.0	1.3
11.	Emphysema	22,249	10.6	1.1
12.	Homicide	20,465	9.8	1.0
13.	Congenital anomalies	14,062	6.7	0.7
14.	Nephritis and nephrosis	8,336	4.0	0.4
15.	Ulcers	7,688	3.7	0.4
	Other and ill-defined	239,584	114.1	12.1

Source: American Cancer Society. *1976 cancer facts and figures*, p. 13.[9]

death that are unlikely to require hospice care are dropped (also excluding both the "other and ill-defined deaths" category and diseases of the heart because many of these deaths are from relatively sudden heart attacks), a total of 507,565 deaths out of 1,973,000 documented deaths in 1974, in the nation, or 25.7 percent of the total remains. Of the death rate of 940.2 per 100,000 population, a need for hospice care is indicated in 241.9 cases.

These figures are necessarily approximate because some patients in certain categories that are not included (e.g., heart disease, stroke, accidents, pneumonia, diseases of infancy) clearly *could* require hospice care, while it is very obvious that some patients in what we might call the "potential hospice care" categories will necessarily die suddenly or in hospitals. The figures do present us, however, with a rough approximation of number of deaths in the general population that are candidates for hospice care.

The most likely candidates are adult cancer patients, although the potential needs for hospice care can reach beyond this one group. There are two reasons for such a limited scope and both reasons are, in the author's view, unfortunate. The first is that the primary and only large source of money for hospice development is the National Cancer Institute. There is no feature of a hospice operation which mandates care exclusively for cancer patients except that, in this country, the National Cancer Institute is likely to be paying for part of that care. That funding agency, because of its exclusive mission, is only interested in care for cancer patients.

DYING CHILDREN

The second unfortunate reason that hospices in the United States are likely to be developed primarily for adult cancer patients is that Americans resist dealing with the terrible plight of dying children. Who among us can contemplate sanguinely the death of children? The current alternative, however, is far worse: dying children are hidden from the view of all of us in the entire society, and even from those, such as physicians, who work in our hospitals. The dying child is a heart-rending sight, especially to doctors and nurses who are trained to preserve life. To them, the dying child represents failure. Visitors may be repulsed by the sight and even the smell of an emaciated dying child. The unfortunate consequence of our repulsion is rejection. Such children are often scattered throughout hospitals, as if spreading out the population of dying children makes each case easier for the rest of us and decreases the probability that any one staff person will have to confront more than one such tragic case at a time. The parents also find it easier to pretend that their children will not die if they are not surrounded by other dying people.

Furthermore, because we hate to see children die even more than we hate to see adults die, and because children cannot refuse treatment, aggressive life-preserving therapies seem to be practiced even more vehemently on them than on adults. Children are completely vulnerable to the psychological needs and whims of their physicians and their parents. They cannot (as many adults learn to do in the final months of life) simply hold up their hands and say: "Stop! All that you have done for me has not worked very well. Many cancer patients, two out of three, are not cured. I want to accept my fate and learn to live well while dying, without the pain and the suffering caused directly by the drugs and the surgery you continue to try on me."

Hospice care for children, then, should be researched. We do not know whether benign and positive modes of care can be developed for dying children in separate programs and facilities. We do not know whether children die easier if they are segregated and cared for separately, in conjunction with dying adults, in conjunction with adults who expect to survive, or with healthy children. Regardless of the theories some of us may hold about which modes of treatment and care are preferable for children, it is clear that the modes that our society has adopted are those that are convenient to parents and doctors, and not necessarily the most beneficial to children.

It may be that only our larger metropolitan centers have populations of dying children large enough to justify the cost-efficiency of separate facilities. If we as a society choose to impose cost-effectiveness criteria on the development of special programs for children who are dying, we may not be able to defend the building of separate facilities.

These reasons constitute an important criticism of hospices as they are being developed presently. Hospices can be designed for all ages, for all categories of dying people. Funding sources and cultural proclivities are limiting the scope of the early hospice programs. We must not continue the tradition of ignoring the special needs of dying children; they cannot be treated as if they are adults. And while we are forced to focus on cancer victims as the primary clients of hospice care, we must distinguish the characteristics of cancer victims from those of other dying people.

DEATH FROM CANCER

It is certainly true, of course, that cancer is by far the leading cause of death among the "potential hospice care" categories, accounting for 69.2 percent of such deaths (and 17.8 percent of all deaths). Cancer sites differ significantly by sex and age of the patient. Geographic region and race also influence the likelihood of different types of cancers.

As Table 5 indicates, during the past quarter-century cancer in males has risen dramatically, while cancer in females has declined slightly. By far the greatest increase for males and females (135 percent and 173 percent, respectively) has been in lung cancer, while stomach cancers have shown the greatest decrease (about 57 percent for both sexes). In males, cancers of the kidney and pancreas have also increased significantly, while cancers of the colon and rectum have declined.[10]

Cancer statistics differ, significantly over race, too. The lifetime probability of developing cancer is about 24 percent in black females and 31 percent in white females, a difference that holds true even though it is generally assumed that underreporting is more of a problem for the black population. In males, however, the situation is reversed. Between 1947 and 1969, the incidence of cancer has risen only slightly in white males, but has risen dramatically among black males, so that cancers of the lung, colon-rectum, prostate, and esophagus now claim many more black males than white males.[11]

Cancer is diagnosed at a stage more favorable for treatment purposes in whites than blacks, and within any stage of the disease, survival rates are significantly higher for whites than blacks. Thus, as Table 5 indicates,[12] death rates for black males are 217, compared with 173 for white males, and 136 for black females compared with 116 for white females.

A dramatic rise in cancer mortality statistics has occurred only for black males, but the control of cancer is more difficult among all blacks generally than among whites. Blacks are developing more cancers, and they have poorer prospects for diagnosis while the cancers are in a localized state. Survival rates are poorer, and death rates are higher for blacks.[13]

Early in 1977 the National Cancer Institute (NCI) released the latest large-scale study on cancer deaths by race, based on death certificate information for 35 types of cancer compiled by the National Center for Health Statistics from 1950 through 1969.[14] Cancer death rates differed dramatically by race, with 189 deaths per 100,000 population for black and Chinese males, 174 for whites, 158 for Japanese, and 100 for Indians. Black females had a death rate of 142 per 100,000 compared with 130 deaths for whites, 109 for American Indians, 91 for Chinese, and 83 for Japanese.

Blacks have a proportionately higher death rate for cancers of the mouth, throat, esophagus, pancreas, lung, stomach, bladder, larynx, cervix, and for mutiple myeloma (a cancer of the bone marrow). Whites have significantly higher rates for cancers of the colon, rectum, breast, ovary,

Table 5
Comparison of Death Rates for United States, 1950 and 1973, for Selected Sites of Cancer by Race and Sex

Site	Race	Males				Females			
		Rate in 1950	Rate in 1973	Change in Rate	Percent Change in Rate	Rate in 1950	Rate in 1973	Change in Rate	Percent Change in Rate
All sites	White	144.7	172.9	28.2	19.5	130.5	115.8	−14.7	−11.3
	Nonwhite	136.6	216.8	80.2	58.7	139.8	135.6	−4.2	−3.1
Esophagus	White	3.9	3.7	−0.2	−5.2	1.0	1.0	0.0	0.0
	Nonwhite	7.0	12.1	5.1	72.9	1.9	3.3	1.4	73.7
Stomach	White	20.4	7.8	−12.6	−61.8	11.1	3.7	−7.4	−66.7
	Nonwhite	28.2	16.1	−12.1	−42.9	14.5	7.0	−7.5	−51.7
Colon-Rectum	White	23.2	23.2	0.0	0.0	22.0	18.0	−4.0	−18.2
	Nonwhite	15.6	18.5	2.9	18.6	16.7	17.3	0.6	3.6

Pancreas	White	7.2	9.6	2.4	33.3	4.8	5.6	0.8	16.7
	Nonwhite	5.8	11.3	5.5	94.8	3.7	7.3	3.6	97.3
Lung	White	20.6	54.5	33.9	164.6	4.4	12.4	8.0	181.8
	Nonwhite	15.5	65.7	50.2	323.9	3.7	12.8	9.1	245.9
Female breast	White	—	—	—	—	24.5	25.4	0.9	3.7
	Nonwhite	—	—	—	—	20.3	24.0	3.7	18.2
Uterus	White	—	—	—	—	19.0	8.1	-10.9	-57.4
	Nonwhite	—	—	—	—	40.6	19.1	-21.5	-53.0
Prostate	White	15.7	15.4	-0.3	-1.9	—	—	—	—
	Nonwhite	19.6	28.3	8.7	44.4	—	—	—	—
Bladder	White	6.1	5.9	-0.2	-3.3	2.6	1.6	-1.0	-38.5
	Nonwhite	4.3	4.6	0.3	7.0	3.0	2.4	-0.6	-20.0
Kidney	White	3.2	4.1	0.9	28.1	1.8	1.9	0.1	5.6
	Nonwhite	1.9	3.2	1.3	68.4	1.3	2.0	0.7	53.8

*Per 100,000 population standardized for age on 1950 U.S. Census Population.
Source: National Center for Health Statistics.

testes, skin, lymph system, kidney, and for leukemia. American Indians, Chinese- and Japanese-Americans all suffer significantly higher mortality rates for certain other cancers. In addition, the incidence of cancers by geographic region was striking. While some of this uneven distribution of cancers by geographic region can be accounted for by the uneven distribution of racial minority groups across the country, it remains generally true that a large number of cancers occur much more frequently in the industrial North and less frequently in the South and especially along the coastal states.

This evidence suggests that environmental factors may play an important role in the cause of cancers. Regional death rate differences from certain cancers are more significant than are racial differences. Access to medical care and exposure to carcinogens are likely to be very important. Although cancer death rates are generally lower in the Southern United States, cervical cancer cases are especially high in some rural Southern areas that are generally poor. (Among black women, who are often among the most poverty-stricken in such areas, the death rates are even higher.) It is possible that racial discrimination in employment may have had the ironic effect of sparing blacks from some important occupational cancer risks in the chemical industries of the Gulf and Southeast regions.

One note of caution should be inserted here. *The Hopeful Side of Cancer,* a booklet recently published by the American Cancer Society,[15] claims that only one in five cancer patients was being cured in the 1930s, and now the figure is one in three. The booklet claims that "in the U.S. alone, 1,500,000 men, women and children are alive, cured of cancer" and the society claims that cancer is "one of the most curable of the major diseases in this country."

Those are dangerous statements if they are not completely true or if they lead to complacency in the general war on cancer. The society's hopeful extrapolations are drawn from only one state, Connecticut, because only that state counted cancer patients in the 1930s. Connecticut has relatively few black residents, it has no city larger than 160,000 people, it is relatively affluent, and it has few people living far from health care facilities.

Other quoted statistics showing the optimistic side of the reality of cancer in this country come from a publication of the National Cancer Institute entitled *End Results in Cancer,* which analyzes the survival rate of cancer patients during the 30-year period from 1940 to 1969. But statistics in this report are based on a sampling of less than 2 percent of the nation's 7,000 hospitals, and of only the hospitals that compiled such data in the 1950s. The sampling emphasizes the larger and best hospitals, with the most modern treatment methods, and those factors may favor better survival figures. In addition, the statistics come from Connecticut, California, and Massachusetts, along with university-affiliated hospitals in New Orleans, Indianapolis, Chicago, Ann Arbor, Charlottesville, and Iowa City. In light of the uneven distribution patterns of cancers by rate, geographic region, and urban or rural setting, it would seem likely that certain biases are built into these unscientifically drawn cancer figures.

These cancer distribution patterns, at any rate, when combined with a perspective on general mortality and morbidity patterns and the status of older Americans suggest that federal coordination and a national planning effort may be desirable if hospice development is to remain rational without unnecessary duplications of service or large gaps in service.

Of the factors that seem to demand more federal intervention in hospice development, the steadily increasing size and political/economic importance of our elderly population is the most compelling. Demographers agree that by the year 2020, there will be nearly twice as many people over the age of 65 (about 43 million) as there are today. This means several things to hospice planners, one of which is that the fiscal pressures on Social Security pension and Medicare systems will grow, probably leading to an increased role for public sector institutions in the health care and general maintenance of the aged population. A growing trend toward institutionalization of health care delivery systems and toward more institutions generally is more likely to lead to the development of a network of hospices across our primary urban areas. Second, lower birth rates will probably result in higher per capita income and less pressure on some governmental income.

While public sector trends suggest that the federal government will encourage the development of hospices and see to their close regulation because of the large governmental interest in the increasing numbers of the aged, the corresponding private sector trends suggest that families may: 1) keep the elderly with them for longer periods of time, 2) be able to afford high quality care for the aged when needed, and 3) demand more outpatient and family-centered care for the elderly than is presently available, precisely the sort of care for the dying that hospices purport to offer. If hospices come to be recognized as a family-centered source of high quality care for the dying and the bereaving, it seems likely that the demand for them will greatly increase during the next several decades. Just as increased education, leisure, and income often result in greater specialization of roles within an industrialized society, so on a smaller scale families that face impending death are likely to find it useful to turn for help and support to specialists in death, dying, and bereavement. These conclusions, which auger well for hospice development during the rest of the century, assume, of course, that hospices will appear in the public mind as centers of high quality care. If the identification with high quality does not take place or is impeded by a mix of various qualities of hospice service across the country, a reliance on hospices may not materialize. Chapters 3 and 4 approach the question of whether hospices are likely to produce the quality of care that will be required by a great many Americans as we move into the next century.

3

The Quality of Dying in America

The complex network of needs displayed by the dying include psychological, cultural, social, medical, and physical elements that are only partially understood by many professionals. Even with all of the attention recently paid to the subjects of death and dying, the voluminous literature on the needs of dying patients has never summarized the numerous research studies or aggregated them into a needs-based model that is understandable and usable by lay people and professionals alike. A descriptive model of the needs of dying people, and of those who watch them die, is important, however, if we are to evaluate the usefulness of hospices and other institutions designed to meet those unique needs.

The status of death and the process of dying in America today may be grouped into two major sections: (1) individual responses to death and (2) institutional responses to death. The former includes all the primarily psychological factors that research has shown to be present in the ways individuals cope with their own deaths and the deaths of others. The latter section comprehends the personnel who manage our death system: who they are, how and why are they recruited for the jobs they do, and how well do they perform their functions in the death system. These descriptions of individual and institutional responses to the process of dying in America help provide an answer to this important question: What type of institution(s) is (are) required to do a better job of meeting the needs of dying Americans?

INDIVIDUAL RESPONSES TO DEATH

General Concepts in the Study of Death

How a person psychologically handles his own death depends, at least in part, on his developmental background, the methods he has used often during his life to handle stress and anxiety, the point in the dying process at which he finds himself at any given time, and the psychosocial environment with which he must contend,[1] according to Kastenbaum and Aisenberg. Whether a person is trying to understand the death of another or the death of himself, he has to develop such complex concepts as absence, abandonment, separation, as well as the fact that each of these concepts when applied to death has a limitless quality to it. The child has a particularly difficult time dealing with limitless absence, abandonment, and separation.[2]

The Plight of Children

Children, because of their limited psychological development, have special problems when they are forced to confront death, either their own death or the death of a loved one. As Natalie Issner puts it:[3]

The child with a malignancy is exposed to many anxiety-producing situations in his total environment, particularly within the hospital setting. Strange, painful procedures, frequent monitoring of bodily functions, tearful or tense facial expressions, secret conversations between parents and physicians, etc., augment his sense of disquietude. The school-age youngster who is acutely ill is especially aware of subtle changes in relationships when he communicates with those around him, and he therefore responds with anxiety.

Children who experience the death of another person also have special problems:

As soon as children become aware of the fact that man is mortal, the fear of death is upon them. Their reactions to an experience with the death of a significant person in their life are influenced by the way their parents deal with it. Deprived children are more vulnerable than those who feel secure and loved. Some children have fears that they have caused the death by disobedience or death wishes at a time of anger.

Conscious efforts are required to help these children, efforts from people with specialized, professional training that is only rarely available to vulnerable children today.

John Schowalter[4] points out that sick children feel anger at parents for failing to protect them and fear that they will be abandoned. If anger predominates, children often become rebellious; if fear dominates, a child may become overly compliant. Parents, too, experience guilt, grief, fear, and anger. Because of the strong relationship between young, dependent children and their parents, it is crucial that parents spend as much time as possible with dying children, but their own affective reactions to death may make this very difficult. Separation anxiety is the dominant reaction of infants to death, and guilt is dominant in preschoolers because illness is often seen as a retribution for bad thoughts and actions. Early school-aged children hold some concept of terminality, Schowalter says, and begin to consider the possibility of afterlife.

Parents of dying children, too, experience major psychological stress:[5]

> Once the parents have been told the child's fatal prognosis, their whole life shrinks. There is routinely a period of denial, after which the process of mourning begins. It is impossible for the parents' attitude toward the child not to change. It is also impossible for the child not to recognize this change. This recognition may not be readily apparent, but the child senses that his parents are distressed and that his relationship with them is different. Although their attention toward him may increase, the perceptive child is also aware of the subtle intensification of feelings that anticipate the process of mourning.

The nature of the marital and parent-child relationship must be discerned by any professional who is called upon to deal with the death of a child. If those relationships are characterized by respect, affection, honesty, well-defined roles, empathy, and tolerance, the management of death will differ substantially from those relationships characterized by hostility, guilt, rejections, overprotectiveness, envy, permissiveness, or harshness.[6] Such topics as initial reactions of children and family members, interim reactions, anticipatory grief, informing the siblings, and terminal reactions clearly require specialized knowledge and even formal training.[7]

Death Fears

If specialized training is valuable when managing death among children, how much more is it valid in dealing with fear, the most common child or adult reaction to death. As Kastenbaum and Aisenberg put it, "fear is the psychological state that is most often mentioned when clinicians or researchers discuss responses or attitudes towards death."

The host of research data on death fears vary in range of subjects from surveys of 1,500 adults to intensive analysis of single cases, and in range of methodologies from interviews and clinical case methods to experimental manipulations, personal diary techniques, the psychological autopsy method, and other multidisciplinary approaches.[9] Fears of and during the dying process, fears of death *per se,* death fears in special populations, death fears and other psychosocial variables (e.g., ambitions, religious affiliation, concepts of sexuality), death anxiety scales, the limits of fear, and various aspects of sorrowing, overcoming, and participating are all subjects that have been studied in the past two decades. It is a reasonable conclusion that high quality treatment of the dying and of those who participate in some way in the death of another requires a thorough familiarity with and understanding of the best available knowledge in the subjects. The currently available body of research, while far from complete and exhaustive, requires specialized training to master well. The studies of death-related concepts available to the average lay person are not adequate to the complex task of meeting the needs of the dying and the bereaved. Death fear is the most common human reaction to death; it is related to many other fears and includes fear of dying, of an afterlife, and of extinction. The etiology and symptoms of death fears are extremely complex.

Previous Personality Factors

The task of meeting those needs includes developing an understanding of the psychological background and history of a dying person and the bereaved. Kastenbaum and Aisenberg note as a general proposition that the selection of coping mechanisms depends in part upon the developmental stage (not the chronological age) of the subject, a point not unlike that which Bernard Schoenberg and Robert Senescu[10] make: "Individual differences in response to the threat of illness, helplessness, disability, pain and separation are based on differences in personality patterns which in turn are derived to a large extent from past personal experiences." Another study notes that delay in even seeking treatment for obvious symptoms of cancer results from such previously developed response patterns as fear of punishment (26.7 percent), fear of death in surgery (15.3 percent), aversion to dependency (13.7 percent), shame or wish to avoid exposure (13 percent), suicidal wishes or extreme resignation (9.2 percent).[11] In still another study, expressions related to death fears were usually expressed as fear of losing a job, leaving the family, dependency, surgery, or as an indication of weakness.[12] People who delayed seeking treatment, analyzed in two other studies, are often the "strongest" among us, those who are autonomous, self-delineated, independent, resistant to assume the role of patient and to "submit" to physicians.[13,14]

It is obvious that staff of various institutions that house the dying can provide a higher quality of care if they understand and appreciate the significant effects of previous personality traits upon the immediate problems of coping with death.

Other Common Death Reactions

Schoenberg and Senescu examine and summarize a number of other common reactions among the dying. Dependency is the first of five typical reactions, for "the patient is inevitably placed in a dependent position which causes him to feel childlike and helpless. Many patients react to this state with resentment since it reawakens feelings of weakness and smallness, and arouses feelings of inferiority and shame."[15,16]

Schoenberg and Senescu consider the expression of anger to be the next common reaction. They write:[17]

Like fear, anger can be an anticipatory response to the threat of pain, damage, or loss of function. In the hospital, the expression of anger is discouraged even more strongly than fear. The fearful, compliant, ingratiating patient is likely to be rewarded, while the angry, demanding, complaining patient often elicits punitive or retaliatory behavior.... To control or hide anger, he may withdraw from all self-assertive behavior and become emotionally inaccessible.

Loss of self-esteem is a third very common reaction to the process of dying that many people have to endure. The authors state:[18]

In general, the factors that contribute most to the reduction of self-esteem are: a) illness and loss of capacity to function; b) loss of the feeling of self-sufficiency and independence; c) fear; d) guilt; e) inability to gain gratification; and f) the individual interpretation of the attitudes and feelings of significant figures (family, physician, and nurse) toward him.

Guilt is another common reaction. Schoenberg and Senescu put it simply and briefly:[19]

The patient may feel guilt over hostile thoughts and feelings as well as overtly angry behavior. An ill patient may view his disease as punishment visited upon him for past sins and indiscretions.

And, finally, many patients experience a distinct loss of pleasure:[20]

A common clinical problem is how to persuade a patient who recognizes that his life span is limited to engage in pleasurable activity. Although modern hospitals have emphasized making physical facilities more attractive, they tend to ignore the patient's personal sources of pleasure. In most hospitals the opportunity for pleasurable activity is usually limited, highly routinized and quite peripheral to the therapeutic program.

Bereavement

The anger noted by Schoenberg and Senescu is a far more common reaction to death than is frequently realized. Rosenblatt, Jackson, and Walsh[21] conclude that "it is not uncommon for people who are bereaved to be angry and even to engage in violent acts," a notion that is supported by the studies of a large number of researchers.[22] In the United States, so-called ritual specialists, such as physicians, clergy, and funeral directors are expected to help to channel and partially resolve feelings of anger.[23] The quality of such channeling, however, is often inadequate and is accompanied by suppressed feelings of anger and aggression.[24] Helping the bereaved deal with anger, then, is yet another area that calls for professional care.

The plight of widowers in dealing with bereavement is especially severe because of the lack of support offered them. Consider the anxiety evident in this report by a widower:[25]

> I expected to be lonely, but never realized just how lonely one could be. Conditions were bearable on the job, but there was little time left after work for daily decisions and planning. Each day I would call to see if the youngest had arrived home from nursery school. Thankfully, each day he had. Also, thankfully, no one realized for six years I left the house unlocked, although other homes in the area were burglarized. A small and excitable dog was always left inside, and he may have been of some help. At least he was someone for the boy to come home to.

The anxieties and stresses associated with widowhood may be linked to extraordinarily low levels of mental and physical health. The death rate of widowers above age 45 is double that of married men in comparable age categories,[26] and the suicide rate below age 45 is highest for widowers. The depressing statistics regarding their psychological health suggest a large-scale need for more professional training and services to help them handle their problems.

Bereavement may be considered as illness in itself because of the complex of symptoms which may become exacerbated and even fatal, whether the bereaved person is male or female. Austin Kutscher points out that despite the bereaved's symptoms, his illness, "in general, is left untreated":[27]

> His state is usually diagnosed from the medical and psychological points of view as a normal response to the circumstances of his situation—until overt signs and symptoms reach pathological proportions. The bereaved, as a patient, requires treatment, especially in the early stages, to prevent a more serious progression.

Kutscher concludes:[28]

> Few teaching or training programs exist which prepare the physician to manage the vicissitudes of grief in medical practice. Recognition of the stages of bereavement, including anticipatory, grief, is important not only for the physician but also for the nurse, social worker, and chaplain.

Kutscher's concerns underscore an important need that hospices may be able to meet, an idea that will be examined further in Chapter 4.

Generalized Modes of Coping with Death

Researchers have not been very successful in combining the most common reactions to death into one coherent model. Shneidman[29] uses five patients dying of cancer as summary examples of various methods of coping with death: The "postponer" wishes not to die and exerts a will to live; the "acceptor" is resigned to death; the "disdainer" is scornful and does not believe death is imminent; the "welcomer" awaits the end of his life with some pleasure; and the "fearer" fights the notion of death.

A wide variety of physical symptoms, including insomnia, lethargy, anorexia, fatigue, and constipation are associated with the depression that often results from the dependency, anger, loss of self-esteem, guilt, and loss of pleasure noted earlier.[30] Even pain, according to Gonda, may be influenced by a person's feelings about his impending death.[31]

The control of chronic pain, while it may have important somatic and psychological benefits, also presents problems to the physician and other professionals who must help the patient manage it. A variety of sedatives and hypnotics are available for various sleep problems, and barbiturates are available with a number of other undesirable side effects.[32] Additional drugs are available for daytime sedative control of anxiety, as well as highly specialized drugs for patients with organic brain disease, states of panic, agitation, increased psychomotor activity, or acute psychotic or manic reactions.[33] Schoenberg concludes that:[34]

> The medication itself may be less important than the manner in which it is given. Having to ask repeatedly for medication is demeaning for patients and undermines the patient-physician relationship. Whenever possible, patients should not be kept waiting for drugs and a program of continuous control should be established. At the same time, the practice of "snowing" the dying patient with excessive medications can be demoralizing since it disrupts his relationships with others and isolates him further from his environment.

Two additional elements of a generalized psychological profile of dying people can also be noted briefly. First, the symptoms of pain and the manifestations of psychological problems may be relative in time. Strauss and Glaser, authors of *Awareness of Dying,*[35] say that such awareness changes day by day and may retrace paths it has already taken. Drastic changes in death perceptions are quite common: "The change may be sudden, temporary or permanent. Or the change may be gradual: nurses, and relatives, too, are familiar with patients who admit to terminality more openly on some days than they do on other days, when pretense is dominant.[36]

The second element of relativity that should be inserted in a profile of dying people concerns the popular belief that dying people pass through several psychological stages in a predictable order. Elizabeth Kubler-Ross published the best known list of stages in 1969, and they have served as the model for much work among dying patients.[37] Kubler-Ross observed that 197 of the 200 dying patients she studied passed through stages of denial, anger, bargaining, depression, and acceptance. But as Schulz and Aderman of Duke University put it, "While Kubler-Ross based her conclusions on information obtained through highly subjective personal interaction with over 200 dying patients, other researchers have attempted to plot the emotional trajectory of the dying patient with more objective methods."[38]

A large number of rigorous tests and assessment devices have been administered to dying people by researchers who have "generally found, in agreement with Kubler-Ross, that most terminal patients experienced depression shortly before death," but the researchers have failed to obtain any consistent evidence that other affect dimensions also characterize the dying patient.[39] The relativity of death perceptions, as well as the relativity of stages of dying, present additional reasons to believe that professionally trained personnel are perhaps most competent to deal with the many complex aspects of the dying process.

INSTITUTIONAL RESPONSE TO DEATH

Physician Management of Death

Are existing medical personnel adequately trained to deal with dying people and the bereaved? Throughout this chapter, the complicated and varied responses to death exhibited by several populations who must contend with death have been explored. Are people in the healing professions, as they are presently organized and trained, sufficiently capable of managing the death process in ways that are both sympathetic and knowledgeable? The overwhelming evidence clearly suggests that they are not.

Jerry Wiener, writing on the responses of medical personnel to fatal illness, summaries some of the major problems that face doctors when confronted with death:

> Central to the choice of medicine as a career is certainly its function in the alleviation of pain and prevention of death. The physician's role is invested with authority and power, with realistic expectations on the part of the patient for care, as well as magical expectations of omnipotence and infallibility. During the course of his education and training the physician acquires knowledge and skills which make it possible for him to fulfill his realistic obligations. When the physician is significantly influenced by unconscious needs for power over illness and death, his care of patients will be inappropriate.

Pediatricians in Wiener's study simply could not agree on how to handle such psychosocial questions as whether parents should be given a diagnosis of a fatal illness, whether they should be accurately informed about prognosis when they ask, and whether parents should be encouraged to assist with the hospital management of their child.

Schoenberg and Senescu conclude that physicians and hospital personnel in general do not often provide the psychosocial care that is most needed:[41]

Care of the dying patient usually induces so much anxiety in health personnel that in many hospitals emphasis is placed on the routine technical aspects of physical care rather than on the development of close interpersonal relationships with patients.

These authors draw the discrepancy most sharply between the care that is needed and the care that is provided when they write:[42]

Terminal patients are frequently avoided by hospital personnel, thereby increasing their sense of loneliness and isolation. Physicians and nurses may avoid conversation or otherwise distract a patient when he begins to discuss death. When the patient feels that hospital personnel are uncomfortable in allowing him to discuss the taboo topic, he will gradually erect his own communication barrier. It is the conspiracy of silence that is most destructive since it tends to separate the dying from the living and offers the patient no opportunity to verbalize his feelings and thoughts, or allow his positive feelings for others to emerge.

Schoenberg lists five reasonable goals in the management of dying patients. He recommends that dying people should be helped to enjoy the best social and familial relationships of which they are capable, that they may be able to cooperate with medical personnel and have measures taken for their welfare, that they obtain the greatest possible pleasure and gratification under the circumstances, that the patient not be caused more distress and pain than is necessary, and finally that the patient be able to maintain a positive self-image and die in a dignified fashion.[43]

Schoenberg suggests that some physicians participate in an avoidance pattern that leaves the patient isolated, an implication that is supported by other researchers, notably Strauss and Glaser:[44]

> The most standard mode is a tendency to avoid contact with those patients who, as yet unaware of impending death, are inclined to question staff members about their increasing debilitation. Also avoided are those patients who have not "accepted" their approaching deaths, and those whose deaths are accompanied by great pain. Staff members' efforts to cope with death often have undesirable effects on both the social and psychological aspects of patient care and their own comfort. Personnel in contact with terminal patients are always somewhat disturbed by their own ineptness in handling the dying.

One of the most cruel consequences of the failure on the part of hospital personnel to confront death-related issues directly and knowledgeably is that some patients are rewarded for "good behavior" while others are not rewarded and may even be punished. Strauss and Glaser also describe this aspect of the way medical personnel treat the dying in blunt terms:[45]

> Staff members do judge the conduct of dying patients by certain implicit standards. These standards are related to the work that hospital personnel do, as well as to some rather general American notions about courageous and decent behavior. A partial list of implicit canons includes the following: the patient should maintain relative composure and cheerfulness; at the very least, he should face death with dignity; he should not cut himself off from the world, turning his back upon the living, but should continue to be a good family member, and be "nice" to other patients; if he can, he should participate in the ward social life; he should cooperate with the staff members who care for him and if possible he should avoid distressing or embarrassing them. A patient who does most of these things will be respected.

What the staff defines as unacceptable behavior in aware dying patients is readily illustrated. . . . Some patients do not face dying with fortitude but become noisy or hysterical. Other patients wail, cry out in terror, complain, accuse the staff of doing nothing, or refuse to cooperate in their medical or nursing care. Perhaps the most unnerving are the patients who become apathetic or hostile and reproachful.

Kastenbaum recently reported on the closely related work of an international ad hoc task force that tried to list the current standards of care for the terminally ill. They described the "good death" in the typical medical facility as one which adheres to these standards:[46]

1. The good or successful death is quiet, uneventful. Nobody is disturbed. The death slips by with as little notice as possible.
2. Not too many people are around. In other words, there is no "scene." Staff does not have to adjust to the presence of family and other visitors who have their own needs and who are in various kinds of "states."
3. Leave-taking behavior is at a minimum.
4. The physician does not have to involve himself intimately in terminal care, especially as the end approaches.
5. The staff makes few technical errors throughout the entire terminal care process, and few mistakes in "etiquette."
6. Strong emphasis is given to the body, little to the personality or spirit of the terminally ill person in all that is done for or to him.
7. The person dies at the right time, i.e., after the full range of medical interventions has been tried, but before a lingering period has set in.
8. The staff is able to conclude that "We did everything we could for this patient."
9. Patient expresses gratitude for the excellent care received.

10. After patient's death, family expresses gratitude for the excellent care received.
11. Parts or components of the deceased are made available to the hospital for clinical, research or administrative purposes (i.e., via autopsy permission or organ gifts).
12. A memorial (financial) gift is made to the hospital in the name of the deceased.
13. The cost of the total terminal care process is determined to have been low or moderate; money was not wasted on a person whose life could not be "saved."

These standards were considered unacceptable by the task force experts, because they clearly did not provide for good medical care in meeting many of the needs of the dying and the bereaved.

Professional Management of the Bereaved

These possible reactions of the dying are compounded in the reactions of family members. One fourth to one half of the physicians and other professionals surveyed by Heimlich and Kutscher disagreed substantially on such common aspects of dying as signs and symptoms of bereavement and whether the bereaved can be expected to experience anger, guilt, impatience or diminished sexual functions.[47] There are also significant differences among the professionals regarding what the bereaved should be told by the physician, what advice and aid they should be encouraged to seek, and even whether remarriage constitutes a major problem of the young bereaved spouse. Some consistency in the advice proffered to the bereaved would be beneficial in treating the illness known as bereavement, but it is obvious that present-day medical practices regarding the bereaved are as inconsistent and variable as practices regarding the dying.

The role that family members can play in providing interpersonal support is highlighted by the research of Dubrey and Terrill.[48] For patients surveyed, family members provided the greatest interpersonal support. Family members and familial relationships were most often thought about when alone, thus emphasizing the centrality of the family and the potential usefulness of the family in providing supportive care. This fact stands in sharp contrast with the practices of most hospitals, which severely limit familial contacts.

Personnel in the Death System

Physicians in the Lead. In our culture the professional most often looked to for guidance during the dying process is the physician. But it may be that physicians are less able to cope with death than other people in the general population. Kastenbaum and Aisenberg describe nine thorough empirical studies which conclude that physicians have an above-average fear of death and often choose their career in order to gain more control over their death fears. In addition, medical training is found to encourage a "counterphobic bravado, a desensitization toward death."[49] If this is true, conclude the authors, "the front line of our death system thus would be manned by volunteers who are more intimidated by the enemy than are many of the civilians behind the lines.[50]

Nurses. But physicians are not the only personnel on the front lines. Nurses, too, are called on to render care and comfort to dying patients, often more frequently than are physicians. A number of studies suggest that nurses, as well as other medical personnel in contact with dying people, often respond in ways that do not meet the needs of the dying patients. They are reluctant to respond to calls from terminal patients and their verbal communication is most often characterized by fatalism ("We are all going to die anyway"), denial, and avoiding the discussion of death. In fact, less than one-fifth of nurses, apparently, are willing to enter into a discussion with terminal patients of their thoughts and feelings.[51] Quint points up a major reason for the deficiencies in nursing care of dying people:[52]

> Educational programs in nursing have not generally provided environments through which nursing students develop the capacity to function effectively in situations which are either personally or professionally threatening. Neither have nursing instructors always recognized the emotional impact carried by certain types of patient assignments.

Other Professionals. While hospital personnel in general play a dominant role in managing death in our culture, other professionals within the death system also have been found to be lacking in their sensitivity to particularly salient issues in death and dying. Funeral directors have come under considerable scrutiny and criticism.[53] Many clergymen have been found to be very dysfunctional when meeting the needs of the dying,[54] and the modern day high priests of our culture, the mental health specialists, have done little work with the dying.[55]

However, Duff and Hollingshead[56] in their lengthy and thorough study of the patients in one hospital discovered a social system that centered on a system of accommodations, and noted that even the physical plant may be constructed to facilitate this system. Staff members usually relate to a patient on the basis of a latter's perceived status in the community. Room accommodations and physician sponsorship also are related to social position, and these factors heavily influence the quality of care.

The distribution of physicians and nurses was found to be directly correlated with patient status. Ward patients were the poorest and had the highest mortality rates. Patients there were confused about symptoms and fearful about illness; they were reluctant to discuss emotional and mental conditions, and physicians indicated an interest only in physical disease. The more seriously ill a patient, the more often both he and the physicians resorted to evasions in their communications. The evasions, which extended to and included the families of dying people, resulted in unnecessary treatment, false hopes, prolonged suffering, lingering deaths, and high expenses, along with unrecorded problems during the bereavement process. Often, all of the people in the core group were complicit in this evasion process, with nurses being influenced profoundly by the example of the physicians.

Cultural Factors

A complex network of factors that make the process of dying in this country difficult for many people to endure with dignity and peace have been examined briefly. From fears of dying and other strong emotions regarding death and bereavement to the clearly inadequate training received by most medical personnel and death specialists, questions remain: Why is the rational management of the dying process in America so distasteful? Why is knowledgeable and sympathetic management so rarely found as to be essentially nonexistent?

Perhaps the deepest reasons for our mismanagement of the death process in America stem from our heritage and our culture, what Kastenbaum and Aisenberg term our "death system,"[57] which constitutes all the thoughts, words, feelings, beliefs, and behavior that are related to death. All societies have developed at least one death system through which they come to terms with death in both personal and social aspects. American society, however, faces a set of conditions concerning death that may be altering our cultural heritage in ways not yet understood. For the first time in human history, our lives are not restricted to an extremely limited life expectancy that had confined most people to an active life only in the years of early maturity. Also new in the historical record is relatively large-scale control over natural forces. In addition, modern human beings have relatively little exposure to and a great deal of isolation from the sight of death. Furthermore, the concept of individualism is now more developed than ever before in human history, and modern humans now stand alone with considerably less support from clan, extended family, or city-state than ever before.[58]

In Kastenbaum and Aisenberg's words, Americans regarding death have become "transposed, isolated, technologized and decontextualized."[59] A considerable number of expert researchers believe that the dead have been expelled as unimportant to the social structure; they are relatively invisible and therefore seemingly less real and less powerful. It is even probable, say some researchers, that our excessive, even obsessive concern with accidental deaths (as witness the feature coverage given airplane crashes and fires in the media, even though such accidental deaths as a proportion of total deaths have drastically declined from the days of preautomobile America) is a mechanism to avoid the inevitability of death and to avoid the fact that 95 percent of us die from "natural causes."[60] Thus we deny that death is within us all; we comfort ourselves by remaining within the child's universe of causality; we pretend that only one type of death is inevitable rather than confronting the fact that we all will die.

Some researchers conclude that in modern, secular America death no longer represents the wages of sin but rather an infringement on the right to life and the pursuit of happiness. Our view of death is related to our view of life, and if the good life is seen as much more carefree than in previous times, concern with death is easily interpreted as an expression of a neurotic personality. Furthermore, we see little point, given our conception of what the good life entails, in learning to adapt ourselves to suffering, deprivation, and frustration.[61]

CONCLUSION

The needs of dying Americans as discussed in this chapter can be summarized in four conclusions that can be used to evaluate hospices. These four statements cover the needs of dying adults, the needs of the bereaved, the special needs of children, and the characteristics of professional personnel who manage the process of death. They comprehend the four main sets of needs that clearly are not met in the American death system today.

Dying Adults

Adequate treatment of dying adults requires a psychological history that establishes level of development, relevant previous personality characteristics, and the means of internalizing stress to which a patient has become accustomed. It requires some knowledge of social and familial relationships, the ways in which those relationships adapt to stress, and the ways those adaptations change or develop over time. The complex etiology and symptoms of death fears also call for specialized knowledge for adequate, individualized treatment. The management of a number of common, pronounced feelings has large-scale implications for the quality of dying. These feelings include dependency, anger, loss of self-esteem, guilt, and the loss of pleasure. These and possibly other strong feelings may be integrated into a number of generalized approaches to the problems of coping with death. These approaches often change over time, sometimes quite quickly, and often include very complex ways of handling pain. The approaches themselves are often very complex and are not easily summarized into stages. It is clear, however, that dying people can experience considerable pleasure and satisfaction from a variety of sources, including their own self-image and familial contacts, and often must be helped and encouraged to do this.

Bereaving Adults

The proper management of bereaving adults requires knowledge of the network of significant specialists who have an impact on the individual's strongest feelings. This network is different from person to person and may vary over time. If adequate support services are not available to the bereaved or if they are not helped to take advantage of them, complex symptoms, which may become exacerbated and even fatal, often become observable. This suggests that bereavement can be considered a serious illness and should be treated as such. Familial relationships may be very supportive for the dying person, and this potential source of strength should be taken advantage of more frequently.

The Special Needs of Children Who Must Deal with Death

The management of children who are experiencing death requires particularly sensitive treatment of fears, nonverbal communications, dependence on adults for healthy concepts of life and death, means of repression, and the effect of the quality of the marital and parent-child relationships upon the child. An awareness is called for of the child's different needs at different levels of development. Treatment of the child's family as it impacts upon the child requires an understanding of how family members, individually and as a group, adjust to stress. The management of children who are experiencing death occurs in a situation that changes over time, and initial reactions of shock or disbelief or avoidance are likely to be quite different from interim reactions that include new adjustments to family members and anticipatory grief. These, of course, are qualitatively different than final or terminal reactions.

Personnel in the Death System

Management of the death process requires personnel who are familiar with such feelings as limitless abandonment, separation and absence, and such concepts as animism, futurity, and constancy. The ways in which these concepts develop over time in any individual are varied and complex. Personnel charged with the management of dying people must be committed to treatment of the entire person, not just a disease, and this includes personality factors, social and family relationships, and a variety of sources of the enjoyment of pleasure, satisfaction, and gratification. While staff needs are often paramount in modern day treatment of dying people, the dying individual, the bereaved, and the significant relationship they enjoy should become the proper units of care. Nearly all personnel in the significant death system are poorly trained to deal with the needs of dying people, and it is likely that the professionals who best meet those needs have themselves adjusted to death concepts and thoughts of their own death. Given the very large and significant reasons why our culture avoids death, it seems likely that only a minority of professionals are sufficiently secure enough to properly manage the death of others.

Discovering whether or not hospices meet the special needs summarized in these conclusions can give us a reasonable measure of the quality of care that hospices may provide.

4

Components of Hospice Care

The first hospices were the early Christian hospitals set up to care for all unfortunates, orphans, the aged, the sick, and wayfarers traveling between cities or to holy places on pilgrimages.[1] Florence Wald of Hospice, Inc., in New Haven, Connecticut, found that one 12th Century hospital in England had the following mandate:[2]

> If anyone in infirm health and destitute of friends should seek admission for a term until he shall recover, let him be gladly received and assigned a bed. In regard to the poor, people who are received late at night, to go forth early in the morning, let the warden take care that their feet are washed and, as far as possible, their necessities tended to.

Wald points out that medical management, comfort, and spiritual care (this last within the religious context of Roman Catholicism) were the three primary objectives of the early hospices. Patients were bedded within the chapel, so that religious participation was easily included in the daily lives of patients and staff.

Three other physical aspects of the early hospices are noteworthy. First, there was a pharmacy in the hospice available to inpatients and outpatients and usable by all citizens of the town. Second, the hospice was located in the very center of the town, immediately adjacent to the market place, so that accessibility of visitors and customers to the pharmacy was easy. Third, there was a peaceful, charming, even beautiful courtyard within the hospice walls, a place in which many patients undoubtedly found quiet and solace.

The picture that Wald presents of the early hospices is neither idealized nor romanticized. A few of the early hospices, scattered throughout Europe, are still operating, and they conform fairly closely to Wald's description. The hospice heritage includes an attempt to integrate purely medical practice with a ministry to the soul, i.e., the provision of comfort to the minds and hearts of patients. An open admissions policy with an emphasis on care to the poor characterized these early humane institutions. They were closely integrated with the surrounding community so that patients and visitors had easy access to each other, and the hospice was seen as serving community needs.

Wald maintains that this heritage has an effect on modern day perceptions of hospice care. As she puts it:[3]

> What has this to do with modern medical care or care of the terminally ill in an age when X-ray therapy, organ transplants, and chemotherapy are commonplace procedures? Hospice care is an attempt to restore the concern for man's spiritual side, as well as retaining modern medical expertise in the management of symptoms caused by illnesses.

Attention to the physical symptoms of a patient, which is the traditional hospital focus of attention, is important, of course, but hospice care goes well beyond that:[4]

One goal of service in a hospice is to provide expert medical management of symptoms, and to comfort always. The second equally important goal is to understand the particular life style of the patient and to help those involved live through this period in a way that gives this style the greatest chance of being fulfilled. For some ... it may be a usual routine and a no-nonsense verbal communication with a mate. For another it may mean being with family and friends as much as they can. For another getting the house in order and making plans for the children will be most important.

Most modern hospitals have space for beds but not for visitors and families, and for the dying person the family offers support and comfort that no nurse or doctor can provide. As Wald puts it, "The hospice defined its recipient of care as a unit of people, the one who is ill, the immediate relatives, and persons in the patient's life."[5]

The hospice also offers care to the bereaved beyond the death of the patient. In a modern hospital, the moment of death is a signal to the patient's family and the hospital staff to part company. In a hospice, however, this is a critical time in which attention becomes focused even more strongly on the needs of the bereaved. Frequent visits are called for with some family members, and while others may need little follow-through, a bereaved person may return for care from the hospice staff at any time.

Another principle is described by Wald as "care and concern for the staff."[6] She draws on her own experiences to define the phrase.[7]

I worked with patients in the home, in the hospital, and in nursing homes, and realized full well the energy which is expended in helping the terminally ill patient. This energy must be replenished if the helper is to sustain his or her capacity to understand, empathize, and respond to situations of crisis and suffering. No helper can bear this burden singly. A doctor cannot be a star, nor can staff exclude the patient or his family from decision making. The worker who cannot accept weakness in himself, or cannot be a receiver as well as a giver, soon finds himself exhausted and bankrupt, or has developed defenses that cripple his humanity and ability to help.

She later describes in a general sense the types of people she tries to recruit for Hospice, Inc.:[8]

> Dr. Saunders has advised us to look for people who have gone through something in their life situations and have come out the other side by having really whipped it and become stronger in the process. We find people who have lost a parent, a child, or a spouse, to be particularly helpful. These are the people who will develop and encourage confidence in patients and their relatives. Bonds between people and one's own internal resources are equally important. The openness and concern for one another is what sustains the hospice family. We need humanists with professional skills who can help by both medical management of symptoms and emotional support.

So if one principle of hospice care involves institutional concern for the staff, another is closely related to it: the recruitment of professionally competent staff who are sufficiently secure in their own internal resources to offer strong support to the totality of the patient, which includes emotional and psychological symptoms.

Yet another principle of hospice care again focuses on the needs of the dying patient; specifically, that drugs and dosages be carefully adjusted for changing symptoms and conditions.

Careful attention to the physical design of the hospice is important, too. A design that promotes independence of movement is desirable, says Wald, as well as one that permits both privacy and company.

> It must be space which is very flexible, which assures privacy, space which can accommodate a crowd around a patient's bed and yet which makes intimate moments possible and pleasurable.

This principle concerned with the physical design is noted by a number of authors as an important aspect of hospice care. Lo-Yi Chan designed the New Haven hospice (as noted in Chapter 6) to have transitional spaces in order to psychologically ease patients into the hospice, with dining rooms, a day-care center, pleasant reception rooms, a sky-lit family room with fireplace and cozy seats, bedrooms that permit patient interaction, and private bedrooms for intimate times with family members, a morgue or suitable body-viewing room, staff lounges, and even a soundproof meditation or screaming room.[10] As Cicely Saunders put it recently. "A building can help ... A good building can make a difference to the backs and feet of the staff," and to the spirits of everyone involved. "Beauty," she added, "is very healing."[11]

One more principle of hospice care noted by Wald involves the integration and incorporation of children into the life of the hospice. A nursery school for the children of both staff and patients is a good idea, she suggests, as are joint meals, snacks, or teas in the garden.

Another important aspect of hospice care is to encourage considerable interaction among the dying patients themselves. Wald proposes:[12]

> Having gone through the same thing, many patients are able to understand and to help their neighbor more than the staff is able to help. And in that helping process they get something out of it.... Patients in my study expressed it beautifully by saying they were concerned about what was going to be happening next, and that it was the fear of the unknown rather than what actually went on, which was difficult to bear.

The hospice concept also encourages the community-based care-givers who have had previous experiences with a patient and the family to continue contact and care, especially at home. Wald points out that it is often difficult to get a patient's regular physician to come to the dying patient at home and that the medical staff of the hospice usually must f ill the gap; nevertheless, physicians, social workers, visiting nurses, and other care-givers can offer important continuing support to the patient and family.[13]

Expert care is multidisciplinary in nature and requires a professional teamwork approach; it may require professional intervention with several institutions in the society. At the same time, the hospice concept ensures that all those affected by the patient's death are considered. This includes the incorporation of family members into the decision-making process even when special education may be required.

Dr. Cecily Saunders[14] of St. Christopher's Hospice suggests that a home care program and the use of volunteers are also important to a good hospice. A home care program can facilitate ease of transition between hospice and home. Volunteers may be used by the hospice to provide both diversity of skills and community contacts. Finally, the hospice, through expert unobtrusive and responsive administration, can provide for excellent recording of the data necessary for evaluation and research so that our knowledge of the dying person's needs may be furthered. At the same time, the hospice is in a unique position to offer educational opportunities to the wide variety of specialists who have contact with the dying.

The major components of hospice care, then, may be summarized as follows:

1. Expert, multidisciplinary management of pain and other symptoms.
2. Easily available personnel and other sources of comfort whenever needed.
3. Reasonable fulfillment of individual life-styles.
4. The provision of care and consideration to all those affected by the patient's death, including the incorporation of family members into the decision-making process, even when special education may be required.

5. Continuing follow-up care for the bereaved.
6. Special care and concern for the staff.
7. Professionally competent staff who are sufficiently secure in their own internal resources to offer strong support to the totality of the patient, which includes emotional and psychological symptoms.
8. Appropriate choices of drugs and dosages, carefully adjusted for changing symptoms and conditions.
9. A physical design that permits independence of movement, privacy, and community.
10. The integration of children into the life of the hospice.
11. Considerable interaction among the dying.
12. Continuity of care to patients and families whenever possible, with care-givers previously acquainted with the patient in the community receiving encouragement to continue contact and care.
13. The capacity for professional intervention in the multifaceted problems that face the dying and the bereaved, including interaction with institutions in the community.
14. Home care and outpatient programs that facilitate ease of transition between hospice and home.
15. The use of volunteers to provide both diversity of skills and community contacts.
16. Administration which provides excellent recording of the data necessary for evaluation and research, as well as educational opportunities for the wide variety of specialists who have contact with the dying.

The question that naturally arises is whether the characteristics of hospices relate routinely and directly to the conclusions about the quality of death discussed in the last chapter. Do hospices, in reality, meet the needs of dying adults, the needs of the bereaved, and the special needs of children? Do hospice personnel fit the unique characteristics of professionals who manage the process of death? The case studies of hospices in Chapters 5 and 6 help to answer these questions. It must be noted, however, that while much of what has been described as indicative of the way hospices operate and will continue to operate in the future, it remains to be seen—and rigorously to be evaluated—to what degree each of the listed components is realized in fact. The list of hospice components as presented here is a mixture of objectives not yet realized in this country and characteristics that have indeed been shown to be achievable in these new institutions. In other words, the most pronounced characteristics of operating hospices, as well as the plans of several hospices not yet off the drawing boards have been taken to construct an archetypal hospice and a model of hospice care. This has been done because hospices are so new to our country. No additional data on actual hospice operations in the United States are available, but the components of hospice care are very likely to be achieved by Hospice, Inc. and probably by other hospices in earlier stages of development.

Another important point to keep in mind when analyzing how hospices meet the needs of the dying in the United States is that the appropriate management of death involves both science and art. Hospice care, in the end, is only as good as the services the staff can provide, and that in turn depends in large measure upon the quality of personnel, the quality of training they have received, the quality of the interactions among staff members, the support the staff receives from the administration, and the relations the staff enjoys with the surrounding community. Certain characteristics of death and dying are dealt with adequately by hospice staff if those hospices are operating as they are intended or planned to operate, and if the best that the professionals have to offer becomes available to patients and the bereaved. Put another way, hospice care, in addition to being a crude science in the sense that it is difficult to prescribe and measure, is also an art because certain aspects of appropriate care cannot be prescribed, predicted, or measured.

While it is difficult to maintain that hospices will have a short-term effect on the cultural characteristics of the death process (although they may have long-term effects through training programs, professional intervention with selected institutions in the surrounding society, and the training that volunteers receive), it seems quite probably that hospices will significantly and positively affect the quality of dying for all those who become clients of hospices.

The strength of hospices lies in the unique and effective way that they meet the special needs of the dying and the bereaved, which are not met often within the existing health care network. If what we know from recent, high quality research about the requirements for good personnel in the death system is applied to the recruitment and selection processes engaged in by the hospices, it seems highly likely that the quality of care that hospices provide, and the responsibility and responsiveness to the dying patient and the bereaving family that hospices are designed to demonstrate will result in a level of care far higher than has previously been available to Americans. The usefulness of hospices will have to be evaluated further as more data become available on the actual operations and the dispersion of effects throughout our society, but at this early point, it is clear that hospices are a positive step in meeting the needs of people.

5

Case Study I: St. Christopher's Hospice

St. Christopher's Hospice[1] opened in Sydenham, England, southeast of London, in July 1967, after 19 years of preparation and planning by Dr. Cicely Saunders and many other committed individuals. Although there are 30 hospices throughout England, St. Christopher's has come to be viewed throughout the world as the prototype of terminal care.

A Board of Directors at St. Christopher's is responsible for policy decisions, although decisions rarely come to a Board vote. Dr. Cicely Saunders is Medical Director, with daily medical care overseen by a Deputy Medical Director. The Matron is responsible for nursing care in the hospice. She is assisted by two experienced nurses who work with the staff and assist in administrative duties. Administrative departments include Domiciliary Service, the Clinic, Study Center, Clinical Research, and Volunteers.

The primary purpose of St. Christopher's is the management of terminal illness. The most notable symptom to be managed, of course, is pain, but there are also nausea, vomiting, breathlessness, incontinence, and anorexia. The staff of St. Christopher's recognizes that they have developed an expertise in the care of the terminally ill and therefore try to admit those patients who will benefit most from being at St. Christopher's. The Admissions Committee, composed of the Matron, social worker, head of Domiciliary Service, and the Admissions secretary, meets daily to review the applications.

St. Christopher's receives about 1,500 inquiries a year and admits between 500 to 600 annually to their 54-bed facility. In selecting patients, the committee considers these criteria: (1) the medical history of the patient, (2) expected length of survival, (3) whether the family can benefit from hospice support, and (4) whether the hospice can help the patient with, for example, specific unresolved problems or symptoms. Other considerations include whether the family lives close enough to enable ease in visiting and what the referring hospital's "reputation" is for terminal care. Patients represent diverse socioeconomic backgrounds as well as a variety of religions.

A patient's admission is of great importance and consequently is carefully planned. The patient is greeted in the ambulance by the Matron. From the ambulance, the patient is helped into a warmed bed and proceeds with the family to the ward where they are met by the Ward Sister (head nurse). The Deputy Medical Director or one of the other physicians arrives promptly and talks alone with the family in order to get a picture of the patient's condition during the preceding few weeks. He or she then returns to talk with the patient, trying to discover which symptoms are causing greatest distress. The admission is a very personal welcome designed to put the patient and the family at ease.

The change in a patient's general condition within a few days of admission is often dramatic. Some patients eat solid food for the first time in weeks, or sleep through the night without wakening, or are able to get out of bed into a chair without assistance. These are small successes, but very important to the patient. Family members also find relief knowing that the patient is well cared for and able to enjoy a few pleasures again.

More than 60 percent of the patients admitted to St. Christopher's Hospice complain of severe pain, which is not infrequently overwhelming. Pain due to advancing cancer is usually chronic, a continuing problem rather than a short-term event. Depression, anxiety, fear, mental isolation, other unrelieved symptoms, and pain itself tend to exacerbate the total pain experience.

The philosophy of St. Christopher's is to prevent pain from occurring rather than to control it once it appears. Analgesics are given every 4 hours, the aim being to match the level of analgesic with the patient's pain, gradually increasing the dose until the patient is pain-free. The next dose is given before the effect of the previous one has worn off and therefore before the patient may think it necessary. This approach, coupled with a sensitivity to the emotional, spiritual, and even financial pain, makes it possible to erase the memory and fear of physical pain.

An analgesic widely used at St. Christopher's is the "Brompton's cocktail," an oral mixture consisting of 2.5 mg (or more) of heroin, 10 mg of cocaine, 2.5 ml of ethyl alcohol (95 percent), and 5 ml of syrup (66 percent sucrose in water) made up to 20 ml by addition of chloroform water. Almost all patients receive a phenothiazine syrup with the diamorphine mixture, to relieve coexistent nausea or vomiting as well as to mask the bitter taste of the diamorphine.

Polypharmacy is the term coined by Dr. Saunders and her staff. Essentially there is little concern for the underlying pathology; rather, the symptoms of the dying patient are of paramount concern. Although pain alleviation is the key to the treatment method, and this is emphasized, extensive drug therapy for a wide range of symptoms is also a core concept, although not sufficiently publicized.

Diamorphine (heroin) is the mainstay of pain relief, and oral medication is preferred. PRN (administer-as-needed) orders are not policy; instead, regular administration of diamorphine is ordered so that patients do not anticipate pain and do not have to wait for medication. They do not wait for the staff to notice that they are in pain, nor must they request medication. Well trained nurses, understanding fully the philosophy of polypharmacy for the relief of symptoms, are given a large degree of choice in administration of dosage since the physician specifies a range of doses permissible in the initial prescription. The nurse uses this latitude of dosage, administered at regular intervals, to meet the clinical needs around the clock. In the same way, multiple drugs with similar effect are used to control nausea, and other symptoms. Thorazine and derivatives are likewise regularly prescribed. For brain metastases and increased intracranial pressure, dexamethasone is used to great effectiveness. The initial prescriptions are supplemented by dosages that may have to be given during the night and are in addition to the list of standing drug orders.

The drugs that patients arrive with are not suddenly discontinued since this might create anxiety. New drugs initially might be ineffective, thereby creating further anxiety and a loss of confidence in the Hospice staff. It is noteworthy that the initial 12 to 24 hours of adjustment to the Hospice often brings about spontaneous relief of symptoms. The initial hours are used to evaluate the needs of the patient. In most cases the activity of travel and transfer aggravates symptoms, whereas the security of the Hospice reception after arrival and the total environment in itself is therapeutic.

The object of polypharmacy is to maintain a functioning individual who is neither in pain nor symptomatic in any other area and who, if able, can be alert to his or her surroundings. When there are obvious signs of death or rapid deterioration, medications may be withdrawn except for diamorphine which is increased in dosage until death. Hyoscine is given to dry up excessive bronchial secretions thus eliminating the "death rattle" that is so distressing to relatives, if not to the patient.

The drug management program at the Hospice is not based on standing orders or benign neglect. On the contrary, it is tightly controlled by daily nurse and physician rounds during which the medication needs and their effectiveness are reviewed in detail, with appropriate adjustments based on the judgments of highly qualified nurses and the evaluation of the medical staff. Patients' complaints and symptoms are sympathetically evaluated and in all instances the benefit of doubt is given to the patient. Concepts such as fear of inducing addiction in the dying patient are irrelevant: a patient in pain seeks relief of pain and, once relieved, usually tolerates a reduction of the dosage. The patient does not suffer the psychological dependence and the acute cravings of the classic drug addict whose entire purpose in taking addictive drugs is a mood "lift" or "high" and whose physiological state is constantly stressed by intermittent, irregular, and in most instances, less than optimal drug dosage. The acute cyclic undulations that drug addicts are subject to are alien to the narcotic regimen of the patient in pain. Similarly, the use of Butazolidine, Chloramycetin, etc. and their possible toxic hematological side effects are of no concern to those caring for the terminal patient. Generally, survival is not sufficiently long enough for toxic reactions or addiction to become real problems in a hospice setting.

This form of medical management avoids chemistries, x-rays, infusions, and intubations, except for urinary catheters if needed. The general policy is not to request autopsy, and only occasionally are corneal tissues obtained.

The focus of the nursing care at St. Christopher's is also quite different from that in the acute hospital setting. In the hospice, the *quality* of life is of primary importance.

Tests and procedures are generally inappropriate; rarely are I.V.'s or transfusions a method of care. Death is viewed as a natural process and is accepted calmly, without heroic efforts to prolong life. Time is spent with the patient so that he or she is kept comfortable and not left alone. The goal of staff efforts and the source of staff satisfaction is the easing of pain and of the symptoms of disease. Because they take the time to consider every complaint, staff members usually are successful in relieving distress. Considerable time is spent in sitting and visiting with a patient in an attempt not only to ascertain immediate concerns, but also to communicate to the patient that he or she is still valued as a person. Hence, the common complaint of feeling isolated and abandoned is heard much less frequently.

Despite the multiple involvements of patients with staff and other patients, the privacy of each patient is respected. Those patients who do not wish to join the activities are left to themselves. Those who wish to remain outside the general activities, or do not wish to speak or be spoken to, use the device suggested by the staff of merely closing their eyes to indicate a desire to be left alone. The philosophic orientation at St. Christopher's is that the total care of the dying patient refers not only to the medical management of symptoms but more importantly to the concept that anything that produces distress or pain for the dying patient or the family is the concern of the Hospice. Hence the total social-emotional-religious impact of the dying patient is managed, including the psychic, physical, and social pain of the bereaved family up to and subsequent to the death of the patient.

Recognizing that the members of the patient's family are under a tremendous strain, the staff actively tries to support them. Although each member of the staff becomes acquainted with the family, the Ward Sister is most closely acquainted with their needs. The spouses of some patients express pleasure and surprise that the staff recognizes them and knows their names, as well as their children who are less frequent visitors.

The bereavement follow-up program for surviving relatives also relies on close acquaintance with the family: the strengths, weaknesses, and need for support are summarized for the "key" person (e.g., spouse, child, parent) related to the patient. The staff determines which people most clearly need bereavement follow-up. These individuals are then visited by volunteers for as long as necessary (generally up to 12 months). The volunteers, selected for this work, meet once a month with the staff to review their interactions with the relative.

An integral aspect of the hospice program is a Domiciliary (Home Care) Service which supports those patients who wish to remain at home with their families. St. Christopher's Domiciliary Service is staffed by an administrator/nurse, two additional nurses with ward experience, and a nurse visitor with psychosocial training. Approximately 80 patients within a 6-mile radius of St. Christopher's can be maintained at home. The hospice staff does not provide nursing care, but they coordinate care with the patient's general practitioner and district nurse. Patients are told to call any time when problems or questions arise.

Patients and families are visited weekly by one of the Domiciliary Service staff. Personnel are not assigned to a particular family since it is found that the patient and family should not rely exclusively on any one staff member. Since 10 percent of St. Christopher's patients are discharged to their homes for various lengths of time, there is a weekly review of Domiciliary patients in order to keep all the staff up to date.

A small clinic is held at the hospice once a week for ambulatory patients. Upon arrival, patients are seated in a circular seating pattern in the waiting room and are introduced to each other. A volunteer is on hand to serve tea and biscuits and stimulate conversation. The physician greets each patient individually, chats briefly, and then proceeds to the examining room. In this informal atmosphere, the patient and family quickly familiarize themselves with the staff, the other patients, and the hospice facility.

There are three different levels of nurses at St. Christopher's: 1) the head nurse who has nursing and leadership experience, 2) a staff nurse who has received formal nursing training and is state registered, and 3) the auxiliary nurse, who has little or no nursing training. Auxiliaries, many of whom are part-time, are trained by working closely with the experienced staff members. Each member of the staff is chosen by the Matron, who makes her decision based on a lengthy interview and her own instinctive responses.

TRAINING AND SELECTION OF STAFF

There is no formal preparation or training prior to working at St. Christopher's. New nurses are closely supervised and are initially assigned to work with an experienced staff nurse until they become fully acquainted with the methods of care. Special training classes for auxiliary nurses are held weekly. There is a 3-month trial period for all staff members. Only 1 week's notice is necessary if a staff member or administrator becomes dissatisfied with the situation. After 3 months, when performance of the staff member is reviewed, he or she is then either hired permanently or asked to leave.

Once a week each ward holds a general meeting that is attended by all the staff, as well as the Matron, the chaplain, the social workers, Domiciliary Service administrators, and a staff doctor. Particular patients are discussed in an attempt by the staff to coordinate all the information and personal interactions. Other problems and issues are raised at that time.

St. Christopher's originated outside the National Health System and is presently supported by both NHS funds, as explained below, and private charitable donations. The hospice staff, consequently, is considered outside the regulatory review of the National Health System but may return to the NHS without loss of benefits.

St. Christopher's recognizes that caring for terminally ill patients is very demanding work and extensive vacation time is allotted. Auxiliary and staff nurses receive 5 and 6 weeks vacation respectively, and the head nurse has a 7-week vacation.

A Director of Volunteers coordinates the activities of over 135 volunteers who serve in three different capacities for a total of more than 600 hours each week:

1. An untrained volunteer assists in nonmedical aspects of care, i.e., filling water containers, tending the plants and flowers, assisting with meal distribution, writing letters or reading to patients, transporting patients or relatives, typing, etc.
2. Some volunteers work as auxiliary nurses and are responsible for such simple nursing tasks as assisting with blanket baths, feeding patients, assisting staff nurses.
3. Professionals who volunteer their time are completely absorbed into the routine. One volunteer physician is responsible for weekend duty twice each month, and a physiotherapist maintains a regular schedule of patients.

Volunteers are specially selected to participate in the bereavement follow-up program.

Screening and selection of volunteers is largely an intuitive process by the director of volunteers, who holds a lengthy discussion with each one and examines his or her reactions to a personal tour through the hospice. Frequently, relatives of deceased patients offer to volunteer but they are generally encouraged to wait from 6 months to 1 year before becoming involved with patients.

St. Christopher's has a firm commitment to education and training. The Study Center serves this purpose where a 4-week multidisciplinary program for students is offered every month except August. After the first week of orientation, the student becomes a member of a ward team and is then directly involved with patient care. Nurses who are new to St. Christopher's are asked to participate in the orientation week in order to gain a better understanding of all the departments within the hospice. They spend time in all the departments of the hospice and with many senior staff members.

Each week the Study Center offers interested professionals and lay people the opportunity to participate in an interdisciplinary group and to learn more about its methods. Student and practicing nurses also have a weekly opportunity to acquaint themselves with St. Christopher's. The staff at the Study Center also responds to requests for presentations at universities in nearby London and at local citizen organizations.

Professional education programs are offered at the Study Center as well as study days for the staff and volunteers. Physicians and nurses may arrange to work or study at St. Christopher's in order to obtain broader experience and training in the care of terminally ill patients.

St. Christopher's has an active program of clinical research that has been concerned with pain relief in advanced cancer patients. Summaries are written on each patient supplemented with careful notations regarding a variety of factors such as symptoms upon admission, unrelieved symptoms, the patient's knowledge of illness, psychological state, description of death, etc.

Many relatives find comfort in an opportunity to continue their relationship with the staff and other patients' families. The Pilgrim Club, which meets once a month at St. Christopher's, is a social get-together that offers support to surviving relatives. The Children's Playgroup functions as a day-care center for children of staff members. Their presence at the hospice lends a cheerful note. Every Thursday morning there is a "bar" for patients, relatives, and staff. This is a lively occasion that is eagerly anticipated by patients and visitors alike. It also offers a patient the opportunity to buy a drink for a favorite nurse or doctor.

Monday is "Visitors Day Off," a time when family and friends are asked not to visit the hospice, allowing themselves and the patient a day of rest. Special activities for patients are planned for Monday afternoon.

The food at St. Christopher's is excellent. Patients select a menu a few hours prior to meal time; appetite and general condition are so variable that it is difficult for a patient to make a decision about dinner in the morning. Every effort is made to cater to personal food preferences.

The hospice facility, designed specifically for terminally ill patients, presents a very airy, light, and open atmosphere. One side of each ward consists of windows, with a view to a busy residential street and tennis courts. Original oil paintings are scattered throughout the hospice and there are flowers and plants everywhere.

Each ward is divided into large bays of four to six beds with curtains for each bed when there is a need for privacy. Each patient has his or her own wooden bedside table for belongings, cards, and other personal items. The patient's bed also has his or her name written visibly on the head railing and every effort is made to personalize the surroundings.

Each floor has a large day room comfortably arranged for visiting, a spacious kitchen where breakfast is prepared as well as midmorning and afternoon tea, a small intimate room for privacy with visitors, as well as two single rooms for patients who do not want to be in one of the bays.

Within the hospice is a large chapel that accommodates patients' beds, a cafeteria, a spacious room for larger gatherings, and a lounge for the staff. Connected to the building is the Draper's Wing, a residence for 16 elderly people who are independent yet in need of some supervision. They have their own activities and regular events and there is some limited contact between the residents and patients.

The grounds of St. Christopher's are landscaped with trees, bushes, flowers, and a goldfish pond with water lilies. There is a large open area where patients can be wheeled out, even in their beds. Visitors to the garden may watch the children playing outside.

St. Christopher's is not part of the National Health Service System, although the NHS does reimburse the hospice for 38 beds; the remaining beds, at $350 each per week, are paid for by private contributions. Gifts total approximately £80,000 per year. Patients are not billed for their stay, although many families make a small weekly donation. The cost of care is below that in a NHS hospital, approximately 70 percent of a teaching hospital on a per bed basis, and about 80 percent of a general hospital in England.

The following tables provide a statistical overview of St. Christopher's operations.

Admissions

Number of Patients Admitted	1975	1974	1973	1972
New patients	604	542	554	480
Readmitted from previous years	7	8	10	10
Total	611	550	564	490

Discharges

Number of Patients Admitted	1975	1974	1973	1972
New patients	47 (8%)	31 (6%)	36 (6.5%)	32 (6.5%)
Readmitted from previous years	3	3	1	5
Total	50	34	37	37

Of the 50 patients discharged, 27 were readmitted (some more than once) and subsequently died at the hospice, 3 died in another hospital, 7 died at home, 13 remained alive through the end of 1975.

Source of Referral, 1975

Admitted from	Male	Female	Total	Percent 1975	1974	1973	1972
Hospital	83	138	221	34.25	36.0	35.0	41.0
Home via Doctor	83	112	195	30.25	25.0	26.0	18.5
Home via Out Patient Clinic	99	130	229	35.5	38.5	38.5	39.5
Other	—	—	—	—	0.5	0.5	1.5
Total	265	380	645	100	100	100	100

Diagnoses, 1975

	1975	1974	1973	1972
Number with malignant disease	595	534	555	480
Number with other diseases	16	16	9	10
Total	611	550	564	490

Primary Site of Malignant Tumor (grouped)

Site	Male	Female	Total	Percent 1975	1974	1973	1972
Gastrointestinal tract	59	99	158	25.7	25.0	26.0	25.5
Bronchus	106	39	145	23.5	22.0	19.0	23.5
Breast	—	104	104	17.0	16.0	16.0	17.0
Genitourinary tract	22	54	76	12.2	16.5	19.0	16.0
Central nervous system	10	16	26	4.2	4.5	1.5	3.0
Ear, nose, and throat	11	10	21	3.5	4.5	4.0	3.0
Pancreas	12	7	19	3.0	4.0	3.0	2.5
Sarcoma	8	8	16	2.5	0.5	1.0	1.5
Melanoma (various sites)	3	5	8	1.2	2.0	1.0	1.5
Miscellaneous	4	5	9	1.5	1.0	2.0	1.0
Unknown	14	19	33	5.5	4.0	7.5	6.5
Total	249	366	615	100	100	100	100

Age Groups in 1975 of Patients with Malignant Diseases

Age (years)	Male	Female	Total	Percent			
				1975	1974	1973	1972
Less than 30	2	3	5	1.0	1.0	0.7	1.0
30–39	6	9	15	2.5	2.0	2.5	1.5
40–49	10	24	34	5.7	9.0	8.0	7.0
50–59	45	63	108	18.0	19.5	18.0	19.0
60–69	102	110	212	35.5	30.5	34.0	35.5
70–79	69	96	165	27.7	30.0	28.0	29.0
over 80	11	45	56	9.5	8.0	8.8	7.0
Total	245	350	595	100	100	100	100

Length of Stay for Patients with Malignant Diseases in 1975

Days	Male	Female	Total	Percent			
				1975	1974	1973	1972
0–2	40	33	73	12.2	14.0	16.5	12.5
3–7	71	73	144	24.2	25.5	25.0	20.0
8–14	48	58	106	18.0	18.0	18.0	18.5
15–28	34	76	110	18.5	20.0	16.5	18.5
29–56	30	66	96	16.0	14.0	14.0	17.5
over 56	22	44	66	11.0	8.5	10.0	13.0
Total	245	350	595	100	100	100	100

One Day Residents in 1975
(24 patients died within 24 hours of admission)

Admitted from	Male	Female	Total
Hospital	2	—	2
Home	10	12	22
Total	12	12	24

Summary of Mean and Median Length of Stay
(in days) from 1970–1975

Year	Male		Female		Both	
	Mean	Median	Mean	Median	Mean	Median
1970	—	—	—	—	34	18
1971	—	—	—	—	29	15
1972	30	12	25	15	27	13
1973	21	9	24	11	23	10
1974	17	9	23	12	22	10
1975	19	9	27	17	24	12

Percent of Main Symptoms on Admission

	Male	Female	Both
Weight loss	71.0	60.0	64.5
Pain	60.0	63.5	62.0
Anorexia	61.0	62.0	61.5
Dyspnoea	54.0	43.5	48.0
Vomiting and nausea	34.0	50.0	43.5
Constipation	46.0	41.0	43.0
Cough	55.0	27.0	38.0
Weakness	28.5	24.5	26.0
Fluid retention	19.0	28.0	24.0
Insomnia	29.0	17.5	22.0
Bedsores	18.5	17.5	18.0
Incontinence	19.0	15.0	17.0
Dysphagia	21.0	11.5	15.5
Hemorrhage	11.0	8.0	9.0
Paralysis	9.0	6.0	7.0
Jaundice	8.0	6.0	7.0
Drowsiness	5.0	5.0	5.0
Diarrhea	3.0	5.0	4.0

Patients Who Did Not Have a Problem with Pain in 1975.

Source of Referral	Male	Female	Total
Other hospital	45	50	95
Via G.P.	19	30	49
Via O.P. clinic	35	48	83
Total	99	128	227

16 of these patients subsequently complained of pain, all but one had acceptable relief.

Patients Who Did Have a Problem with Pain in 1975

Source of Referral	Male	Female	Total
Other hospital	38	79	117
Via G.P.	48	65	113
Via O.P. clinic	60	78	138
Total	146	222	368

All but 6 patients obtained good relief from their pain.

6

Case Study II: Hospice, Inc.

Hospice, Inc. is the first American hospice. Its own statement of "What is Hospice" describes its founding philosophy:[1]

> We care for those suffering from advanced cancer or similar disease. We plan to show this concern in a program designed to meet the physical and spiritual needs of those, of all ages, who are unlikely to recover from illness. These needs can be met with skilled medical and nursing care, in the use of every scientific means of relieving distress and controlling pain. . . .
>
> This specialized attention focuses on the family as the unit of care. The unique needs of relatives will be our concern as well as the direct welfare of the patients.
>
> We maintain that this can best be achieved by providing the finest available skills of the medical, nursing and health-related professions, together with available community resources. Our aim is to provide a creative approach to meet the total health needs—physical, psychological, and spiritual—of each patient and family.

Hospice, Inc. in New Haven, Connecticut, is the off-spring of Florence Wald, a nurse at Yale-New Haven hospital who has spent much of her time with dying patients during more than the past decade. She produced a study of the terminally ill and in the late 1960s began to gather around her others who were concerned with the quality of care offered to the dying in the New Haven area. Her group wrote a second study of a more interdisciplinary nature including diaries of patients and caregivers.

A group of founders then united around their vision of what care for the terminally ill should be. The founders' group included Ms. Wald; Reverend Ed Dobihal, Director, Department of Religious Ministries, Yale-New Haven Hospital; and Drs. Morris Wessel and Ira Goldenberg of the hospital. They began a planning process to translate their vision into the reality of meeting the death-related needs of the New Haven community.

St. Christopher's Hospice was the prototype for what a hospice should be, with three differences between two hospices: (1) Hospice, Inc. is multi-religious or nonsectarian while St. Christopher's is primarily, but not exclusively, Anglican; (2) Hospice, Inc. is exclusively for the terminally ill, but St. Christopher's has a wing for the elderly; and (3) the drugs used for pain relief are different and Hospice, Inc. does not use heroin.

Most of the planning group spent time living and studying at St. Christopher's in London. They felt that experiencing a functioning hospice would be crucial to the development of plans for an American institution. Hospice, Inc. has adopted the principles of care already demonstrated in the English model. The visits to St. Christopher's also served an important inspirational function for them as they started their unique project in the United States. Dobihal wrote in the July 1974 issue of *Connecticut Medicine*:[2]

One of my dying friends in the Hospice in England said, "You know it's good to be in this place where I belong. Where I feel welcomed. Where people care—even love me. A place where people have time to share with me. They're never too busy for a smile, a word, or to sit down and hold my hand, even cry with me. So you've come all the way from America to learn from us. Well, go back, and if you don't have places like this, start one for people like me." I heard her request on behalf of others, pray to God daily to help us to meet it, and share it now with you.

The hospice planning group was originally affiliated with Yale University. In November 1971, the hospice incorporated itself with a nonprofit, tax-exempt status and formally severed its ties with the university. The decision to become independent was based on two financial issues and two ideological interests. Practically speaking, the hospice as a part of Yale would have to compete for funds with everyone else at the university. In addition, they already knew that they wanted to build a separate facility and, according to Yale University regulations, that would mean that for every dollar of operating costs, 50 cents would have to go to Yale.

One of the first decisions the group made was that they wanted Hospice, Inc. to be identified with the New Haven community rather than the university because of the importance of community support for such a project. Being independent established their community priority, therefore, as well as removed them from constant conflict with the value system of Yale-New Haven Hospital, which was quite different from what they wanted in a hospice.

From the very inception of Hospice, Inc., its planners have been aware of its function as a demonstrational and educational center in the United States. As such, they have struggled hard to keep it a very "pure" representation of the hospice concept. Huge amounts of time, energy, and money have gone into virtually every aspect of high quality terminal care. By March 1976, Reverend Dobihal was able to report that the hospice movement had taken root and that he had received requests from no fewer than 36 communities across the nation asking for help to set up hospice-type programs.[3] The planners of Hospice, Inc. have been acutely interested in careful, thorough development of America's hospice prototype.

The original planning task force for Hospice, Inc. was made up of 150 individuals, some from medical and related professions and others interested primarily in the community. The original Board of Directors numbered nine people plus staff members. The board now has been enlarged to 18 members to include more nonmedical expertise of a nonmedical nature that is necessary for management, fund raising, and governmental liaison. The board represents some of the wide variety of backgrounds and skills they can draw upon.[4]

The task force outlined for itself and others who planned to establish hospices a suggested program for the development of any hospice:

1. Define the relevant gaps in the health care system.
2. Design a program that will best fill that gap.
3. Stress the uniqueness of the hospice program.
4. Educate the community, and especially the medical community, about hospices.
5. Establish a smaller group to work out the specifics of the program and its implementation.

Education was found to be an enormous part of the task of development. Without the support of the medical community, Hospice, Inc. had no chance for approval from the Connecticut state health commission, but physicians had to be convinced of the effectiveness and value of such an institution. The health commission turned down their petition twice before they finally accepted it. One key to acceptance was "expert testimony," or, oncologists and psychiatrists. At the start of the hearing, two-thirds of the members of the commission were opposed to Hospice, Inc.; in the end, their approval was unanimous.

Community education was also crucial to the success of Hospice, Inc. A large staff of volunteers is necessary to the functioning of a hospice because of the variety and extent of services that are required by patients and families. Community groups and individuals are essential for these services. *Friends of Hospice* in New Haven was organized to do volunteer work, to raise money, and to publish a monthly newsletter. Clergy from the greater New Haven area have had a significant role in the development of Hospice, Inc., and their support and contacts have been important.

In addition, it was vital that Branford residents not feel that a "death house" was invading their neighborhood. In another neighborhood, which was known to oppose the hospice, one resident proclaimed, "I don't want my children molested by those dying patients."[5] The image of the dying as perverse had to be countered directly.

Hospice, Inc., through publicity and one-to-one education, has made itself a community project with broad-based support. At the last state health commission hearing, 400 people showed up to express their support for what Hospice, Inc. was trying to do. Community organization work had produced an impressive list of endorsements.[6]

In January 1972, Hospice, Inc. received a $10,000 grant from the Commonwealth Fund, a local foundation. They proceeded to apply for more grants, to set up task forces, and to establish work schedules. The task forces they first developed were the following:

1. Home Care—to develop a home care program to begin actual patient care as soon as possible.

2. Facility Planning—for longer range planning for an inpatient institution and model hospice.
3. Finances—fund raising for all projects as well as calculating expenses and possible fee scales for the new hospice.
4. Community Relations—to enlist community support and implement Hospice, Inc.'s role as a model for others.
5. Professional Relations and Research—for the education of health care workers, evaluation of the project, and development of medical expertise in the area of pain relief.

The task forces were made up of members of the Board of Directors, staff, and outside people.

Hospice, Inc. has received a significant portion of its funds from private donors, including one anonymous check for $34,000. But most of their funding has been from these foundation grants:

Commonwealth Fund	1972–76	Planning and development
Connecticut Regional Medical Program	1972–73	Research
Ittleson Family Foundation	1973–74	Planning and development
Henry J. Kaiser Foundation	1974–75	Community relations
National Cancer Institute	1974–75	Home Care
New Haven Foundation	1972	Planning and development

New York Foundation	1974–75	Planning and development
Sachem Fund	1973–74	Home Care
Van Ameringen Foundation, Inc.	1973–74	Home Care
National Cancer Institute	1976–77	Home Care

One of the first decisions that the planning team had to make was what population Hospice, Inc. would service. In order to maintain its community base, they chose to narrowly define geographic boundaries as one criterion for selecting patients. Nationally 349,000 people died from cancer in 1973. In Connecticut, in 1970 alone, 4,650 people died from cancer, 280 from polio and multiple sclerosis, and 475 from other degenerative nervous system disorders. As of 1970, there were 5,403 patients in Connecticut with terminal illness who might have benefitted from specialized treatment of the type Hospice, Inc. offers. The proposal submitted to the state health commission estimated that there were 1,100 patients and 3,300 close family members in Hospice Inc.'s catchment area who could benefit from specialized care. The facility will care for approximately 696 patients annually, or 60 percent of those who need it. The catchment area is defined as the New Haven area and the surrounding towns of West Haven, Hamden, North Haven, East Haven, Branford, Bethany, Guildord, Madison, Newington, Milford, and Woodbridge. In this planning region in the period 1969 to 1971, 70 percent of cancer patients died in hospitals, 20 percent of cancer patients died in convalescent homes, and 10 percent of cancer patients died at home. In the period March 1974 to March 1975 the breakdown by towns of the patients and families that Hospice, Inc. has cared for was

New Haven	31
West Haven	11
Hamden	10
North Haven	5
Branford	4
Bethany	3
Guildord	1
Madison	1
Newington	1

Hospice, Inc. subscribes to the same principles of care being advocated and practiced throughout the hospice movement. Foremost is the principle of the family as the unit of concern. A major portion of hospice care is preventive medicine, that is, caring for the survivors so that they too do not become ill. For the dying patient, hospice care means control of the symptoms and pain of the disease and alleviation of fear. As Hospice, Inc. describes it:

These principles include a comprehensive, coordinated program of home care and in-patient care. Particular medical expertise in pain control, the management of nausea and other symptoms, maintenance of alertness and mood will be stressed. Pharmacological consultation and research will be important. Expert nursing care will be given, but in addition, nurses will be specifically trained, and given the time, to attend to the needs of the patient and family. Social work, psychiatric consultation, clergy services, and volunteer activities will be offered to support patients and families and to include them in an on-going living process designed to maximize their valuable contribution and participation.

These concepts have application in general health care, but nowhere are they more important than in terminal care. In the process of dying and bereavement, it is vital that relationships are lived out and concluded as productively as possible. Families will be included as important members of the Hospice team, whether the patient is at home or in the in-patient facility.

Hospice, Inc. has outlined three essential components of quality care to the dying and their families: home care, outpatient services, and an inpatient facility. The Home Care Service has been in operation for more than three years and is already serving as a model for such services nationwide. With money from the Sachem Fund of New Haven, the Van Ameringen Foundation of New York, and, most especially, the National Cancer Institute, the Hospice Home Care Team established as its goal: "To extend the period of time in which patients can be safely, comfortably and inexpensively cared for outside of a hospital or other in-patient facility."[9]

From March 1974 through June 1976 Hospice, Inc. cared for over 220 patients in the Home Care Program, 167 of whom had died by the end of that period. Of these, 47 percent died at home. The research department of Hospice, Inc. estimated that approximately two weeks were cut from the average hospital stay of those Home Care patients who died in hospitals or nursing homes.[7]

Additional criteria for care by the Hospice Home Care Program are the following.

1. The diagnosis must be cancer. This decision was made because the skills of the Home Care team are basically oriented to cancer care and because the program is funded primarily by the National Cancer Institute. When the program develops and expands, care will be extended to patients with other degenerative diseases.
2. The consent and cooperation of the patient's primary physician is a prerequisite. That physician *must* continue to serve the patient throughout the entire illness.
3. The prognosis must be limited (viewed in terms of weeks or months rather than years). The staff is trained to work with patients in advanced stages of malignancy. Those who are admitted to the program generally have a prognosis of approximately three months of life.

4. There must be a primary care-giver in the home—a spouse, friend, or family member. This person must live with the patient. The hospice staff spend a great deal of time teaching these care-givers how to take care of their friends or relatives; that care must be available 24 hours a day. Care from experienced, committed people is essential in this situation, and it must always be available.

Age is not a criterion for care: 60 percent of those cared for by Hospice, Inc. are under 65. The oldest patient was 88; the youngest patient in the Home Care program was 19.

Hospice Home Care is the primary source of care for its patients. The Home Care Program assumes responsibility for the care of the terminally ill cancer patient and works alongside the patient's previous doctor. The Home Care Team contracts with a Visiting Nurse Service for daily care in the home. Hospice staff are not able to visit all patients every day. Nurses visit at least twice a week and a doctor once each week. Volunteers and social workers visit in the homes more frequently.

A unique and important aspect of the Home Care approach is that the team is available 24-hours a day, 7 days a week. Should any crisis occur it can be immediately resolved by the staff. A hemorrhage in the middle of the night need not be complicated by a panic-ridden trip to a strange hospital that may not be equipped to handle the problem. Instead, a doctor is at the patient's bed in minutes with help. Patients never feel alone or abandoned. Help is always available.

With this kind of care, patients can stay in their homes with their families and among the people and things that they care about, as long as they wish. And help is available to the family members who must care for the dying patients as well as resolve their own grief and loneliness.

THE STAFF

The staff of the Home Care Team consists of one full-time physician, two full-time Registered Nurses, three part-time Licensed Practical Nurses, a half-time social worker, a director of volunteers, two secretaries, and a consulting clinical pharmacist. The full-time physician, Dr. Sylvia Lack, came to New Haven from St. Christopher's and most of the rest of the staff have studied, visited, or worked at the hospice in London. This interdisciplinary team approach is considered essential to quality care:[10]

> Every Tuesday, the Home Care Team meets to discuss the patient/families. This meeting includes the doctor, the Director of Volunteers, the nurses, the social worker, outside professionals who may be concerned with a particular case, and the Home Care secretary who has the vital job of taking initial patient referrals and receiving calls each day from Hospice patients and families.
>
> A patient may receive a doctor's visit any time during the week, Thursdays are reserved for "Roving Clinic." On that day, Dr. Lack visits patients and families as a follow-up to the Tuesday meetings. Some visits may be to a bereaved family member, or to Hospice patients who are spending time in an area hospital or nursing home.

Selecting staff for such a project had to be done with great care. Florence Wald made these comments about hospice staff:[11]

> The human qualities each staff member needs and the capacity of persons to relate to one another presents a more elusive problem in developing staff. Dr. Saunders has advised us to look for people who have gone through something in their life situations and have come out the other side by having really whipped it and become stronger in the process. We find people who have lost a parent, a child, or a spouse, to be particularly

helpful. These are the people who will develop and encourage confidence in patients and their relatives. Bonds between people and one's own internal resources are equally important. The openness and concern for one another is what sustains the hospice family. We need humanists with professional skills who can help by both medical management of symptoms and emotional support.

At the same time, the selection process had to weed out people with a mission or cause that might narrow the patients' options, such as newly bereaved people, or people with overly rigid religious convictions.

When interviewing for Home Care nurses the selection committee developed the following criteria for applicants:

1. The nurse must have a good, solid nursing foundation and experience, preferably in gerontology or oncology.
2. The nurse must have psychodynamic skills.
3. Flexibility is essential. He or she must be able to cope with stress and to handle unpredictable events. The nurse must not have a fixed idea of *how* someone would cope with death.
4. Candidates for nursing positions are interviewed by several staff members representing different perspectives.

The nurses see their role as threefold:

1. They supply pain and symptom management. They perform the initial assessment of pain level and a careful evaluation of the patient's response to treatment.
2. They teach the family basic nursing care. They show the family how to give medication and how to help the patient with rehabilitative exercises.
3. Nurses lend emotional support to the patient and family through the period of bereavement.

"The nurses may visit a family once a week or three times a day. Each visit may vary from a half hour to three hours. They make their visits over a 16 hour period during weekdays, and are on call 24-hours a day, 7 days a week. The goal of the Home Care nurses is to be there when their patients need them most."[12]

The selection committee was able to find staff that met both professional and humanistic criteria. Some examples:

Dr. Sylvia Lack did her medical training at St. Bartholo-mew's Hospital, London University. Before going to New Haven, she worked for two years in a joint appointment at St. Christopher's and St. Joseph's Hospices in London.

Sister Mary Kaye Dunn, R.N., was a bedside nurse and head nurse with St. Mary's Hospital in Minnesota, which is affiliated with the Mayo Clinic. She had exten-sive experience with patients in advanced stages of can-cer.

Joan Craven, R.N., was one of the founders of Hospice, Inc. She is a clinical specialist in oncology nursing. She pre-viously held the position of Director of Service Rehabili-tation with the Massachusetts Division of the American Cancer Society.

VOLUNTEER PROGRAM

The volunteer program, as noted earlier, is an essential component of the Home Care Team. Volunteers are care-fully screened through a series of interviews with various staff members and then are accompanied by the staff to the patients' homes where they are watched and evalu-ated. The staff later discusses the volunteers and how they feel about their ability to handle their jobs. If everyone agrees that a volunteer is sincere, humane, flexible, and competent, he or she is given a 10-hour orientation course and is then able to do volunteer work. There are over 40 trained volunteers now working at Hospice, Inc.

Each patient and his or her family presents a variety of needs that call for volunteers with both professional and nonprofessional skills. Each volunteer is individually and carefully matched to hospice activities according to skills, interests, and available time. In the Home Care Program lay volunteers are providing companionship, friendship, transportation, shopping assistance, bedside sitting, or just an extra pair of hands.

In addition, six volunteer Registered Nurses have been incorporated into the program by accompanying a Hospice, Inc. nurse on rounds. These volunteers are especially useful for patient companionship because they are trained to note changes in conditions and symptoms. Family members feel more confident about leaving a patient at home for a while if they know a nurse is present. All volunteers work directly with the nurse in charge of a case. They report back to the nurse regularly.

PAIN CONTROL

As noted several times, pain control is a primary goal of good hospice care. Each hospice develops its own pharmacological approach toward pain relief, but the similarities outweigh the differences. Dr. Lack points out to patients that 50 percent of cancer victims do not experience pain, that pain cannot be assumed to be something that must be suffered, and that pain control should start when pain is only mild. A patient should not have to be in agony to get relief. Dr. Lack's basic viewpoint is that pharmacological pain control is successful only if it is considered in the perspective of other pain (spiritual, emotional, etc.).[13] The most common problems of dying patients are pain, nausea and vomiting, constipation, diarrhea, anorexia, and anticholinergic effects such as dry mouth and urinary retention.

At Hospice Inc., a mixture of pure morphine and water[14] is employed for pain relief. Dr. Lack feels that patients can manage well without heroin. They administer the narcotics in a liquid preparation because it can be titrated more accurately; the proportions of solution can be found that will produce the desired effect without oversedation.

Narcotics are always given with phenothiazine-compazine. This mixture potentiates the activity of the narcotic so that less morphine can be used. Nausea and vomiting from the narcotics are prevented by the use of the antiemetic. The mixture also tastes less bitter than straight morphine. Compazine, in addition, is a mild tranquilizer which helps alleviate the anxiety associated with pain. If this anxiety is severe, Dr. Lack may add benzodiazepines (e.g., Valium) to the mixture.

For one who has chronic pain 24 hours a day, a hypnotic (flurazepam) may be used to get the patient through the night. Elavil is often used in this instance but only in very small doses. It must be used with great care with the elderly in whom it sometimes causes confusion and disorientation.

The goal of titrating narcotics is to find the gap between pain relief and sedation. When the narcotic is introduced, the patient will appear sedated, but this effect will wear off in a few days. For a patient with severe pain, Dr. Lack often starts with a heavy dose (20 mg) of morphine. Once the pain is under control, the dose is reduced by 5 mg every three days until the pain returns. The patient is then maintained at the lowest dosage level that will prevent the pain from recurring. For those patients not in severe pain, Dr. Lack starts with a small dose of morphine and increases it by intervals until there is pain relief. Experience with narcotics in both New Haven and England has shown that people do not escalate dosages; they reach a plateau.

This method of pain control requires considerable effort and exactitude. It also requires more physician time and pharmacological expertise than is available from many doctors. Dr. Lack follows this approach because it prevents either oversedation or undersedation. If patients are either in pain or drowsy, they cannot function to capacity; they cannot "live until they die."[15]

At present, Home Care is given at no cost to the patient family; Hospice Home Care operates under the previously listed grants. Efforts are being made to determine what the cost to the patient will be when the grants have run out and the program is self-supporting. In addition, efforts are being made to enable Hospice, Inc. to collect payments from Blue Cross, Medicaid, and other insurance programs.

Two case histories from the Hospice, Inc. Home Care Program illustrate the Hospice approach:[16]

In May 1973, E. C., a retired Navy warrant officer from Branford, Connecticut, learned that he had cancer of the prostate. By last July, the pain had blossomed and was "eating him alive." When the family doctor pronounced the illness terminal and suggested a nursing home, E. C. recoiled at the idea, and so did his family. "But the boys were going to pieces," recalls Mrs. E. C. "We couldn't stand seeing him suffer."

At that point, many families would have given up and surrendered the patient to an institution, to die in a drugged stupor or in pain among strangers. But today 57-year-old E. C. strides about his own house free of pain and sharing fully in the life of his wife and two sons for however long he has left. E. C.'s escape from the nursing home was due in large part to a new health-care organization in nearby New Haven called Hospice, which furnished a doctor and an array of nurses to counsel the family, monitor the patient's drugs and provide boundless emotional support.

... During a recent interview in their Branford, Connecticut home, E. C. and B. C. spoke of the support they have received from Hospice during E. C.'s fight with prostate cancer.

"Without this help from Hospice he couldn't have come along like he is now," said Mrs. C. "Here he is living and participating in life the way people would, instead of being a vegetable in a bed."

D. K. spent his last months in a rented hospital bed in the middle of the tiny living room of the apartment he shared with his wife on the third floor of a three-family home in a blue-collar neighborhood of New Haven.

D. K., a 76-year-old Ukrainian immigrant, died November 6 of cancer of the esophagus. He refused steadfastly to be hospitalized.

With his daughter-in-law, I. K., translating his Ukrainian into heavily accented English, D. K. explained on a recent evening that "he don't want to go to the hospital, and he knows they are not going to help him any more in the hospital. He say he want to die at home. . . ."

I. K. added "He's not afraid to die, like he said. But he needs at least something to help him with the pain. And that's what you people help him with," she said to Dr. Lack, "the pain."

The doctor, sitting beside D. K. on his bed, asked that he describe what his pain was like when he first was visited by Hospice workers a few months ago.

"It's like a fire inside," translated I. K., "if somebody put a hot iron on your hand, on your skin, that's the pain he feels inside."

But D. K. was being given morphine at such a dosage that he no longer felt the pain. He was no longer lying in a fetal position, a hot water bottle clutched to his chest, staring into space, moaning in his own private hell.

"The goal in the home care program at the moment is to achieve a situation where pain is no longer a problem," Dr. Lack said.

Hospice, Inc. planners intended from the conception of their planning process to include inpatient care for those who needed it. An inpatient facility would specialize in care for those who are not able to benefit from intensive treatments offered at acute hospitals but who are too ill to be looked after properly at home. Also, it would benefit those whose families, wearied by prolonged nursing, need a rest themselves. Such patient/families need many non-medical services that hospitals do not offer.

Planning such a facility required a longer developing process than initiating the Home Care Program. Every aspect of good hospice care had to be carefully and thoroughly examined if Hospice, Inc. was seriously to fulfill its adopted role as a model in this country.

The hospice building committee considered a number of well-qualified architects and, after much debate, chose Lo-Yi Chan, of Prentice and Chan, Ohlhausen. They chose Chan partly because he had never designed a hospital, but especially because he volunteered to spend time at St. Christopher's if he received the assignment. In December 1973, Chan went to London for two weeks. For the first time in his marriage he took his wife on a business trip because they both knew it was going to be an emotional experience they should share. They came away with a changed perspective on death and dying that enabled Chan to return to New Haven and design a therapeutic environment with unusual concern for the feelings of patients and families.

The proposed 44-bed hospice will consist of two V-shaped patients' wings, each attached at its apex to one long service and administrative spine which will also house the Home Care Program. Chan has paid particular attention to providing "transitional spaces"—ways to prepare people before they confront an anxiety-ridden situation. Anterooms will ease people into situations they do not want to confront. Windows and spaces will provide escape valves for visitors, patients, and staff alike.

Antianxiety treatment begins outside the hospice. The glass-walled staff dining room and the day-care center playground will be placed facing the street. People walking by or approaching the building will not see an ominous death house. They will see instead a warm, open place, with children playing, and mobile patients enjoying the fresh air.

Chan designed the entrance to look professional, yet friendly, with one entrance for everyone including patients, visitors, family, outpatients, and staff. Thus Home Care patients transferring to inpatient status will not suddenly have to use a new side entrance. Everyone is welcome. Patients arriving by ambulance will also use the main entrance and will be transferred to a bed in the reception room. People will not be given the sense that they must be hidden. Admissions will be by appointment so that a bed and chart can be waiting for the patient's arrival.

For visitors, the entrance to a patient's room presents a critical place and time. Tension is high and the fear of walking in on a macabre scene is great. Therefore, each 22-bed wing will be approached through a sky-lit family room with a fireplace and comfortable seating arrangements. This space will be soothing and comforting.

Hospice design intentionally concerns itself with sense of community rather than a sense of privacy. Although government regulations call for 60 percent single-bed rooms in new hospitals, an exception permits Hospice, Inc. to have 90 percent four-bed rooms.[17] Interaction of patients, families, and staff are crucial to making Hospice, Inc. work. (Private rooms prevent patients from talking or helping each other through their illnesses.) There are four private rooms with double beds available. These are primarily intended for married patients who should be able to continue to enjoy sexual relationships if they wish; some will just want the emotional security of sleeping together. Private rooms will also be used for patients who are disruptive, disfigured, or who have extremely large families.

In order to prevent guests, patients, and staff from getting in one another's way, Hospice, Inc. has a unique layout—a double corridor plan.[18] Rooms are arranged in rows with corridors on either side. On one side will be a private corridor with bathrooms, supply rooms, sinks, dispensary, etc. On the other side will be a social hallway with a greenhouse facing the patios. It will be wide enough for patients to have their beds moved out to visit with family members.

The greenhouse windows will be the room windows. Wards will have no walls and no doors, just low partitions. The partitions will give a sense of privacy while allowing the nurses to watch patients closely and giving patients the sense of community. This will combat the loneliness and sense of isolation that so many terminal patients feel. The facility averages 1,000 square feet of space per bed as opposed to nursing homes, which average less than one-third of that area. Natural light will be used as much as possible, not only because it is more healthful, but also because it accentuates the passage of time in a palpable way. It ties the patient and family to the knowledge of outside life and its rhythms.

The removal of a person who has just died presented a major planning problem.[19] Area undertakers were vehemently opposed to the inclusion of an in-house morgue in the plans. The building committee was as adamantly in favor of such a plan. They stressed the need to confront death right away, for families to be able to view the body, to make the death "real" right there in comfortable, familiar surroundings. Not viewing the body can have serious effects on those who mourn. When a patient dies at Hospice, Inc. the curtains are drawn around the bed and the other patients in the room are told of the death. The body is prepared and then the private corridor is emptied and the body taken to a special viewing room. The homey, nonfuneral viewing site is a two-room suite designed to accommodate fear of the dead. Intentionally long and narrow, the suite allows family and friends to approach slowly from great distance and to view the body only from the anteroom if they desire. A comfortable chair welcomes anyone who would like to stay with the body for awhile. The dead person is on a familiar, home-like bed and there is a ledge with plants next to the bed so that people can avert their eyes if they desire. This is another example of the painstakingly careful planning that has gone into the Hospice, Inc. facility.

Much attention has also been paid to the needs of staff in this type of institution. The tension and strain of the emotional interactions taking place might be counterproductive. The staff will have separate dining areas and lounges as places to get away with each other. Chan also designed a meditation or screaming room. It is a small room, in neutral tones, lit only by a skylight. It is a soundproof retreat where staff can go to think or to let out tension. It will be a calm, bland area for reenergizing.

Hospice, Inc. will also have a day-care facility for staff, volunteers, visitors, and patients. Staff members will be able to visit and play with their children during their shift. Everyone's spirits are raised by the sight and sound of children playing nearby. Doctors, nurses, social workers, psychiatric workers, volunteers, and religious workers will be able not only to consult with one another but also to relax together and give each other support.

Every effort will be made to maintain the life-style of the families of patients. Relatives and friends will be able to visit, cook special meals, decorate the room with objects from home, etc. Patients will be encouraged to participate in family decisions: ties will not be broken, but strengthened. Children will be welcome and day care will be provided if parents need time alone. Visits from favorite pets will be allowed. Hospice, Inc. is designed to be the most supportive atmosphere possible for those who are experiencing death and dying, for patients, family, and staff to grieve together, and to give strength to those who go on living.

FUNDING

Hospice, Inc. purchased 5.9 acres in Branford, Connecticut, as the site for their inpatient facility. They found the site and a donor of the purchase price in early May 1974.[20] On June 11, 1974, the Connecticut Commission on Hospitals and Health Care approved their plans and the Branford Planning Zoning Commission approved a zone change so that Hospice, Inc. could be built in its residential neighborhood. It is located near an elementary school and a Catholic church. The March 1975 estimate for total cost of the facility was $3.6 million. They hoped to raise $360,000 in the New Haven area and $3,240,000 from state and national sources.[21] Estimates of costs of various parts of the facility follow:

Land Purchase	$ 114,000
Building and Grounds	$3,280,100
Community Support Space (family living room, reception rooms, cafe, chapel, child care center, staff retreat space, craft room, dining room)	$ 830,000
Medical Service Areas (diagnostic radiation room, pharmacy, laboratory, physiotherapy suite)	$ 98,000
Inpatient Care (bed and bath spaces, living/dining rooms, conference room/patient study, green house corridor) Total for two patient wings	$ 71,000

The planners estimate the per diem rate for patients at Hospice will be $108.00. This compares well with the $207.39 per diem rate at nearby Yale-New Haven Hospital. Hospice, Inc. anticipates serving 700 patients per year. Costs are estimated on the calculated assumption that patients/families will need an average of 15 home visits and will need an average of 21 days of inpatient care (Table 1).

Table 1
Estimated Per Diem Cost Comparison in Dollars

Facility	1973	1974	1976	1977
Yale-New Haven	161.21	171.69	194.73	207.39
Hospice, Inc.	83.95	89.41	108.27	108.00

Raising the money to build the hospice facility is still the single largest problem facing the organization. Appeals for funding and publicity about Hospice, Inc. goals have been disseminated nationwide. Foundations have made grants for specific projects necessary for establishing the program. The Hearst Foundation gave $20,000 for construction of an examining room. The Commonwealth Hospice donated $25,000 to cover costs of developing formal relationships with other health care components in greater New Haven.[22]

While raising money has been a continuing problem, other problems are of interest also. Particularly important are the problems Hospice, Inc. has had with government and state agencies. Two cases in point are the issues of four-bed rooms and approval by the Commission of Hospitals and Health Care.

As noted earlier, government regulations by the federally sponsored Health Planning Organization (HOP) call for 60 percent single-bedded rooms in new hospitals. The philosophy of community at Hospice, Inc. required 90 percent four-bedded rooms to foster communications and peer support. In order to have wards, Hospice, Inc. has to call them intensive care units. But by regulation, they must have all beds visible from a single point. That was not possible in a situation demanding space and some privacy. Finally, after much haggling, an HOP relaxed the last regulation.[23]

Licensing the hospice was a major battle that necessitated three hearings before the Connecticut Commission on Hospitals and Health Care. Hospice, Inc. was finally licensed as a chronic disease hospital, but there were three major reasons that licensure was denied the first two times and all of them showed some naivete on the part of Hospice staff.[24]

1. Hospice staff did not know state politics, and did not know that the state health department director was opposed to licensing chronic disease hospitals. In addition, an influential member of the commission represented the nursing home industry, which was vehemently opposed to Hospice, Inc. because it would take their clients.
2. Community education had not been utilized to bring pressure to bear on the committee members. At the last hearing about 400 community people showed up to support Hospice, Inc. and present petitions signed by thousands more. Expert testimony by physicians and other professionals was also utilized.
3. At the first two hearings, the staff did not present hard financial data. For the last hearing they included three-year operational budgets, cash flow plans, how much money they expected to borrow, projected number of patients, average number of days as inpatients, per diem rate of Hospice, Inc., etc.

Having learned from their two rejections, Hospice, Inc. staff put the same thorough approach they used in planning the facility to work in negotiating with state agencies. They then had to approach the federal government and private insurance companies to resolve the issues of third part payments—Blue Cross, Medicaid, etc.[25]

A study conducted by the Hospice, Inc. research staff and included in their proposal to the state commission examined sources of reimbursement for 923 patients who died in Yale-New Haven Hospital from October 1, 1972, through September 30, 1973. Of that total 210 patients died from cancer or neurological diseases, roughly the type of population Hospice, Inc. can expect to serve. For 192 of these, inpatient care was reimbursed as follows:

43.4% from Medicare
9.7% from Medicaid
29.0% from Blue Cross
14.3% from insurance or self-payment
3.6% from other (military, medical program, research money, mother and child program, etc.) From this and other information, Hospice, Inc. estimates that 45 to 50% of their operating expenses will be financed by Medicare. The Projected Operating Budgets for three years, as included in the report to the commission, are shown in Table 2. The projected revenues from inpatient care and home care, respectively, are shown in Table 3.

Planners at Hospice, Inc. have made some of their research and their work available to other groups trying to start hospices across the nation. The New Haven hospice is unique in the United States, and, as such, serves as a prototype for this kind of institution. The planned facility seems as close to ideal as possible and the staff is likely to

Table 2
Projected Operating Budget for Patient Services

1976–1977	$1,441,507
1977–1978	1,758,960
1978–1979	1,869,148

Table 3
Projected Revenues from Two Types of Care

	1976–1977	1977–1978	1978–1979
Inpatient (89%)	$1,283,002	1,565,474	1,663,542
Home Care (11%)	158,505	193,486	205,606
Total	$1,441,507	$1,758,960	$1,869,148

be excellent. But most importantly, the almost evangelical drive of the hospice's founders appears determined to make quality care for the dying and their families a reality in this country. They are acutely conscious of the prototypical nature of their endeavors. They expect that hospice planning groups across the nation will be spurred by their efforts. Major issues they have encountered in hospice development include community relations, professional relations, licensing, staffing, facility planning, and finance. It is quite possible that the experience of Hospice, Inc. planners in these areas may help many of the approximately 90 other hospice planning groups to proceed more quickly with their own efforts.

7

Case Study III: Strong Memorial Hospital— A Failure to Start a Hospice

The Cancer Center at the University of Rochester's Strong Memorial Hospital in New York is a good example of the difficulties hospice planning groups can encounter. Strong Hospice is worthy of study for another reason, too, because it represents an alternative to the models established by St. Christopher's and Hospice, Inc.; Strong was an attempt to start a hospice within a hospital.

There are at least nine reasons for establishing hospices within existing hospitals. Obviously, the argument *against* such a move has to do with the antithetical nature of the two institutions. Hospices properly may be seen as an alternative to and criticism of the social, medical, and physical environment afforded patients in traditional hospitals. Success and failure in hospices are indicated by the quality of death, not by the life and death dichotomy often seen in hospitals. Nevertheless, there are nine important reasons for establishing hospices within existing hospitals.

1. There is no absolutely necessary, or even theoretical, reason why a separate wing within a hospital could not provide high quality hospice care to patients who are acknowledged to be dying.

2. Hospices as separate facilities are likely to be more expensive than when established as part of a hospital that adheres to the principles of hospice care, if for no other reason than that certain economies of scale are available to the larger institution.

3. The nation's hospitals have too many beds. This is a chronic condition recognized by hospital planners and health care specialists nationwide. Most American cities have more hospital beds than demand warrants, thus increasing the costs of all hospital stays. In most cities (and Rochester is typical in this regard), approval by federally sponsored health planning agencies for new beds in a new facility is virtually impossible to obtain. The conversion of existing hospital beds to new uses, such as in a hospice, is more economically justifiable and practical.

4. Hospitals are an important focus of economic resources devoted to health. Quite simply, planners may be more successful in establishing hospices when they appeal to the boards of existing hospitals than when they try to obtain donations from outside sources, many of which are already locked into a tradition of channeling health-related contributions to the local hospital network.

5. Hospices offer a kind of patient care that is often inadequate or missing in hospitals. As such, they represent a way to work within and change the establishment by changing the care available in hospitals.

6. People who want to change the attitudes and skills of physicians and medical personnel who work with dying people can achieve quicker, more uniform, and more efficient results by working with existing person-

nel, in close proximity to them, rather than by isolating themselves in a separate facility.

7. No matter how large the network of hospices may eventually be, some people will die in hospitals. Those people deserve the same high level of quality care delivered to dying patients everywhere. Hospital personnel still should learn to deal with and minister to the needs of the dying.

8. Many communities in the country cannot afford to support a hospice as a separate institution. Rochester, New York, because it has a critical mass of people (300,000 in the city and over 700,000 in the surrounding county) can afford to support a separate hospice with finances, personnel, and sufficient patients. Nearby Ithaca, Binghamton, Elmira, and Corning, to name just a few cities, are probably too small to build and maintain separate hospice facilities. Families should not have to travel to distant hospices in larger cities. Smaller communities can provide convenient access to hospice care by implementing the Strong hospice-hospital model.

9. Hospices as separate facilities contribute to the increasing specialization of the American medical system that has increasingly come under attack. We now have special units for heart attack victims. Specialized facilities may be justified in this instance, but the question remains as to what criteria can establish the need for new medically isolated facilities every time a separate patient population is defined by the planners.

The history and operations of St. Christopher's in England and Hospice, Inc. in New Haven make strong counterarguments to each of the above points. As this chapter will indicate, there are problems with the Strong approach. The financial resources and personnel required by a hospice may be available at a given hospital, but that is not a guarantee that those resources will be allocated to new uses or that important staff members will be sympathetic to a new allocation.

The Cancer Center in Rochester is a widely acknowledged, high quality facility for the treatment of cancer in western New York. The facility was established as a research, educational, and patient-care model by the National Cancer Institute and is still largely funded by it. The center coordinates activities of oncologists throughout the county but has a special relationship with Strong Memorial Hospital, where it is located. Their Oncological Surgery Department is widely respected and used by patients from all over western New York. It is inevitable, therefore, that many patients are dying at Strong at any time, and that no matter what the caliber of treatment, many patients can no longer be helped by aggressive therapy.[1]

In May 1973, Bradford Patterson, Associate Director of the Cancer Center and practicing oncological surgeon, first acknowledged that dying patients at the center were not being treated in a manner that reflected their condition. He admitted that this failing was the fault of physicians who could not or would not accept death and whose treatment of the dying was, therefore, inappropriate. In a memorandum to the Division of Oncology, Dr. Patterson said:[2]

> As it is, we all have widely varying techniques for handling terminally-ill patients, stating that it depends on the patient, the family or family physician. Actually it depends most of all on the attitudes, personality and traditions of the physician-in-charge. I suggest that we develop our own standards based on experience and thoughtful consideration. These guidelines would help us to confront families, teach students and live with our ethical and moral decisions.

His first proposal was to terminate such aggressive treatments as drugs, blood products, and radiation therapy for those patients who clearly were dying and instead to use drugs for the relief of "pain, anxiety, sleeplessness, and thirst."[3]

Patterson's concern initiated discussions among physicians and nurses at Strong Memorial regarding the humane treatment of the dying, about "permitting" a patient to die rather than continuing aggressive therapy, and about determining what the needs of the dying might be. Dr. Patterson began to pursue with others the idea of hospice care for the Cancer Center.

Patterson's next steps were to find resources to support a person to work on the hospice concept, and to concentrate on building support for the hospice idea within the hospital and in the wider community.

Initial response to the hospice concept varied widely, from disapproval to unqualified support. A clergyman suggested that medical personnel were not equipped or able to provide the services needed, that "the primary focus of anyone's activities should be in his own field." From within the hospital, however, came ideological support. A core group of interested, motivated professionals began to coalesce, although none was willing or able to take on primary responsibility for developing the hospice concept further.

Patterson found the right person in Claire Ravizza, who had a strong interest in improving care for the dying, and was eager to develop a hospice program. Patterson hoped to get funding for her to begin immediately at Strong. It ended up being a full year, however, before funding was found to hire Ravizza.

The decision was made to apply for funds from local foundations rather than to try for larger foundations or federal grants. Several foundations were approached, but hopes were largely pinned on the Davenport-Hatch Foundation in nearby Penfield, New York.

With the expectation that the money would be forthcoming by October 1974, Patterson sought funds for the summer from the Euthanasia Educational Council in Rochester, stating:[5]

> Our primary interest is in seeing to it that patients in the University of Rochester Cancer Center not only get aggressive therapy while they are salvageable, but also get optimal care when dying. We feel the need to learn more about helping to make the dying process easier on patients and families. We know that students (nurses, physicians, theologians) need instruction also. Therefore, we feel that a 'resource' which might consist of in-patient units at one or more hospitals and also an out-patient office or 'person' is a necessity. It would not be necessary to limit the facility to cancer patients.

Despite letters of support for the application from the Euthanasia Educational Council, the Davenport-Hatch Foundation denied the request for funds for the Cancer Center.[6]

Next, a proposal was submitted to the local Monroe County Cancer and Leukemia Association. Funding was sought for a feasibility study to explore three sets of questions:[4]

1. Assuming the need for a hospice in the Rochester area, what form should it take? An allocated bed unit in one or more hospitals? A separate facility? A central office providing counsel and financial support for individual beds as needed in each hospital?

2. How would this community resource be staffed and funded? Are there private monies available for such a deserving local cause? What about Blue Cross and other third party carriers?

3. What reception would a hospice have among patients? Doctors? Health planning agencies? Could general support be anticipated or would the fear of "mercy killing" have to be dispelled by public education.

The funding sought was minimal, mainly to pay for the services of Claire Ravizza:[7]

To investigate the feasibility of establishing a hospice in Rochester, we wish to employ an available person, who has not only worked in community planning, but has studied the related problems of physicians' attitudes toward euthanasia.

It was June 1975 before partial approval of that grant was received. The Monroe County Cancer and Leukemia Association (MCCLA) funded the feasibility study up to $13,-675.

Claire Ravizza began her one-year grant by working to determine the need for a Rochester hospice. Through interviews and research on death statistics in Monroe County, she determined that malignant neoplasms (cancer) were the second largest cause of death in the county in 1974, accounting for 1,036 deaths.[8] She found that home care agencies in the city were treating a surprisingly large number of cancer patients. Of a total of 1408 patients treated by the Home Care Association in 1973–1974, 116 were discharged because they died and 161 were admitted to a general hospital as terminal.[9]

A survey of head nurses at Strong Memorial Hospital revealed that, in a one-day survey of 296 beds at Strong Memorial, 18 patients were terminal cases and could be expected to live for fewer than three months.[10] Nurses estimated that 16 of those would benefit from hospice-type care; two would not because they were on life-sustaining machines. All the head nurses voiced support for a hospice:[11]

We are not emotionally equipped to handle needs of dying patients when we are faced with so many demands of the 'curable' patients.

We are too busy to even begin to help the families.

Physical care needs of other patients are so many that there is no time left for dying patients. We are aware of what we are not doing for the terminally ill, but it doesn't seem likely that there will be any change.

Many of us are not comfortable with death, and would welcome the opportunity to receive training in working with dying patients."

Many of the nurses could not accept the fact that they had terminally ill patients on their wards,[12] a problem that was repeated wherever Ravizza tried to gather data:[13]

The biggest problem that I ran across in trying to get hard core data was that nobody, really, identifies the terminally ill as a population. In other words, only two nursing homes in Rochester offer what they call 'end stage' care for cancer patients, and only one of those could say how many were admitted for that purpose.

With her estimates of the number of terminally ill patients, the next step was to determine how many would actually use hospice-type care. Clearly, while hospice care meets the needs of many dying people and their families, other patients may not be interested in those services. Since home care is a vital part of this program, determining the actual number of beds needed to accommodate patients is difficult.

As part of the needs assessment for the hospice, Ravizza interviewed dying patients and bereaved families. She found that:[14]

Family members repeatedly emphasized their conviction that an alternative to an acute hospital bed or a nursing home is needed for dying patients.... Attention to details, 'proper care,' insufficient medication, and loneliness of the patient were cited as deficiencies encountered by the families. We did not find one family who was satisfied with the total care given the patient; few of the families received emotional support through the crisis.

One of the family members interviewed was a nurse whose mother was dying. She repeatedly asked doctors to let her mother die, but they insisted on aggressive treatments which only increased her pain. Her mother at one point said, "When all this flesh is gone, maybe then they'll let me die." Family members stayed with her mother at all times because they felt the care she was receiving was inadequate. One evening, they overheard a nurse comment, in a very disapproving and contemptuous tone, "They've been having a wake in there for a week."[15]

After determining the need, the next step was finding out what community resources were available to meet those needs. Discussions were held first with the voluntary, nonprofit home care agencies—the Public Health Nurses and the Visiting Nurses. On a preliminary basis, talks centered on selecting nurses who wanted to work with terminal patients and who would be good candidates to receive extra training in hospice care. The home care agencies, of course, might retain control over selection of their staff, but these specially trained nurses would be available when the hospice had a terminally ill patient at home.

Ravizza continued to explore community feelings regarding a hospice and available community resources by visiting every agency whose activities might be involved, from the Council on the Aging, to all the cancer agencies. Besides sharing information, her visits allayed community fears of the new project and produced added advice.

Early in this endeavor, a decision was reached to exclude pediatric patients from whatever facility was developed unless it was exclusively for home care. Neither St. Christopher's Hospice nor Hospice, Inc. accepts children as patients. The reason in Rochester was that the pediatric population would always be too small and that it would be overwhelming to a child to be with so many adults. In addition, the pediatric oncologist at Strong Memorial felt that they did a good job with their dying patients, and he might be opposed to a hospice if it was to include children.

Under consideration, then, at Strong, were: 1) a separate facility, 2) a hospice unit within an existing facility, 3) a home care program, 4) scattered beds within an existing facility, 5) a resource person to act as a patient advocate for dying patients.

At the end of the first six months, Ravizza and Patterson recommended to the Monroe County Cancer and Leukemia Association (MCCLA) that a hospice be developed within an existing hospital. They based their recommendation on the following reasons:[16]

1. Many human and physical resources are readily available in hospitals; by locating a unit there, one avoids unnecessary duplication.
2. Patients and families are at present oriented to a hospital setting when advanced disease is present. If they were moved out of a hospital at this stage they will feel (and will be) abandoned by their doctors.
3. A hospice unit would round out the spectrum of care in a general hospital, providing care at the end of life which is as skilled and specialized as that provided at the beginning of life.
4. A hospice located within a hospital affords opportunity to educate students, medical staff, and other professionals about the importance and need for specialized care of dying patients. The hospice approach would also benefit terminally ill patients within the particular hospital who were not in the hospice unit. The hospice unit need not be established in only one hospital. As the concept gains acceptance most general hospitals will be receptive in significant ways.

5. The hospice unit with an accompanying integrated home care service would prove more economical than our current system of care. Families feel more secure caring for a patient at home when they know there is a highly trained staff who may be consulted at any time; the result is that more patients remain at home to die. When a patient enters a hospice, unnecessary procedures are omitted also resulting in savings to the community.

The deciding factor was that there were surplus beds in Monroe County and there was virtually no way to get approval from the state for new beds in a new facility. There also was no category under which to apply for government money for a new facility that would fit the hospice description. Chances of getting a new category approved were negligible.

Their plan for the next six months was to begin a process whereby a hospice might become a reality in the Rochester area. Professionals who deal regularly with dying patients (nurses, physicians, social workers, clergy, and others) were contacted and found to strongly support the hospice concept.

In addition, Ravizza attempted to strengthen relationships with other hospitals in the area. When it was clear that the hospice would be located in an existing facility and that there were several hospitals and nursing homes interested in becoming the site for such a facility, competitive tensions appeared for the first time. Two hospitals besides Strong (St Mary's and Highland) had extra beds for which they did not want to lose certification, and both were very interested in the hospice concept as a possible way to fill those beds. But Patterson had funded Ravizza and the message to her was to keep the hospice at Strong.[17] Information was shared with other facilities, but Ravizza's time and planning went to the Cancer Center at Strong, as she worked out the final draft of the feasibility study.

THE FEASIBILITY STUDY

The final draft of the feasibility study included all the data compiled by Ravizza regarding the need for a hospice, a proposal for a hospice for consideration by Rochester area hospitals, and a detailed one-year budget estimate for a hospice unit. The study, which bore Patterson's and Ravizza's names, had several conclusions similar to their MCCLA reports, as well as several new ones:

1. There is need for an alternative form of care for terminally ill patients in Rochester.
2. There is support in the community for the development of a hospice among physicians, nurses, social workers, administrators, and clergymen as well as laymen.
3. Preliminary reports from Hospice, Inc. of New Haven, Connecticut, indicate that hospice care may permit significant savings over acute general hospital care. When their facility opens, the cost per day will be $109, as compared to $200 per day for acute hospital care in the greater New Haven area. It is recognized that some of this cost may reflect lower construction costs, but a substantial amount also must represent lower daily "charges" for intravenous treatment, antibiotics, etc.
4. There are compelling reasons to develop a hospice unit at a general hospital, rather than in a separate facility. Many human and physical resources are already available in a hospital, so unnecessary duplication can be avoided. Patients and families are oriented to a hospital setting, particularly when advanced disease is present. A hospice unit can round out the spectrum of care in a general hospital, providing care at the end of life which is as skilled and specialized as that provided at the beginning of life.
5. Payment for daily charges in a hospital-based hospice is available from the usual insurance sources.

6. Start-up funds may be available from local foundations or private individuals who are interested.

7. The first hospice unit would serve as a demonstration resource to the community by working with other hospitals and long-term care facilities to assist in establishing additional programs or hospice units elsewhere.

The study also presented the six major components of Strong Hospital Hospice.

Palliative Care

Expert medical and psychosocial management of dying patients is the primary purpose of the unit. Only those tests and procedures that are of utmost concern will be ordered, and pain medication is liberally dispensed. Families are encouraged to participate in patient care.

Staff

Physicians, nurses, social workers, clergy, psychologists, etc., will work closely together to provide care that is best suited to the patient and family. The ratio of nursing personnel to patients is high (1:1) since nurses give generously of their time to patients instead of being involved with aggressive therapy. Volunteers will also be trained to assume a major role.

Interaction of the Hospice Unit with the Hospital

Education and training are important functions of the hospice. However, access to patients must be carefully regulated. Nursing and house staff need not be assigned to the unit as an obligatory aspect of their training. The hospital staff will inevitably benefit from the hospice experience, and hospice staff will be available for consultation regarding other terminal patients.

Environment

The physical environment of the unit is an important aspect of the care of the patient; the goal is to develop a positive, home-like atmosphere of welcome and confidence, as well as a sense of community.

A hospice unit needs considerable autonomy as regards visiting and patient activity. Visting hours should be open; family may stay overnight when the patient becomes critical. Children of all ages are encouraged to visit; there should be a constant merging of patient, staff, visitors, and children, and a minimum of rules and regulations.

Home Care Service

This essential component of any hospice program supports and coordinates community resources, enabling patients to remain home as long as possible. Special personnel will provide consultation and support to patient and family, supplementing that currently provided by home care agencies. Experience in New Haven, has shown that with this service there is a significant increase in the number of patients who die at home.

Administration

The Hospice Unit should function as a distinct entity reporting to the director of the hospital. A medical director and unit administrator will be responsible for operational decisions. An advisory committee composed of key hospital personnel and community members is needed to develop the unit.

An important element of the feasibility study was the one-year budget estimates for a 16-bed hospice unit (Table 1).

FUNDING FALTERS

In addition to the major, descriptive study, a grant proposal for submission to the National Cancer Institute for funding of the demonstration and training portions of the hospice plan was prepared.[18] The proposal included an outreach program that could offer other hospitals and long-term care institutions in the region information regarding hospice care and other resources available for the dying. Community education was also proposed for the second year of operation.

The training portion of the unit would include inservice education for nurses and physicians stressing the interdisciplinary team approach, new techniques of nursing care including symptom management and pain control, and discussions of the importance of emotional, spiritual, and social support of dying patients and their families. A training program of hospice volunteers would also be developed. While the National Cancer Institute could have funded part or all of the proposal, in October 1976 they rejected the entire contract.[19]

The funds for Claire Ravizza's study from MCCLA expired in June 1976. Another proposal to MCCLA was written requesting funding for another year for Ravizza, but when officials of the Cancer Center decided to approach MCCLA to fund an unrelated project, the hospice development proposal suddenly was shelved and the Cancer Center came up with the money to keep Claire Ravizza on staff.

Table 1
First Year Budget Estimates

Functional Title	Number Needed	Time (%)	Salary ($)
Inpatient Services			
Medical Director—responsible for medical management of patients	1	50	15,000
Coordinator/Administrator—responsible for daily operation	1	100	15,000
Nurse Practitioner—responsible for nursing management	1	100	15,000
Nurses (R.N.)—responsible for total patient care and family support	10	100	11,000 (110,000)
Social Worker—support patients and families, assist in home care patient management	1	100	13,000
Psychiatrist/Psychologist—assist staff, families and patients with psychological needs	1	20	8,000
Chaplain services—for spiritual and emotional assistance to patients and families	1	40	5,000
Administrative Secretary—performs clerical and administrative duties	1	100	9,000
Patient Care Assistant—housekeeping and daily maintenance activities	1	100	7,300
Medical Specialists/Consultants	1	as needed	3,000
Volunteers—assist in all phases of the inpatient unit and home care service	7–10	part-time	0
Dietitian	1	as needed	
Physiotherapist	1	as needed	
Pharmacologist—consultation regarding pain control and symptom management	1	as needed	
Subtotal			200,300
Total Inpatient Services plus fringe benefits			230,000

(Continued)

Table 1   (Continued)

Functional Title	Number Needed	Time (%)	Salary ($)
Home-Care Services			
Nurse Practitioner (Community Health)—administration and patient care	1	100	15,000
RN—patient care and family support	1	50	6,000
Volunteers—same personnel as those on unit	2–3	part-time	0
Subtotal			21,000
Total Home Care Service, including fringe benefits			25,000
Total Salaries and Fringes			$255,000
Supplies			
Hospital stores			13,750
Sterile supplies			2,750
Laundry			8,000
Pharmacy			2,000
Office supplies, phone, etc.			700
Subtotal			27,200
Estimated Total 1-Year Operating Costs			282,200

Tensions between Ravizza and the hospital began to increase as she questioned the extent of the hospital's commitment to a hospice. She demanded a public statement from the hospital, but Dr. Patterson urged restraint, arguing against pushing the hospital too hard. Ravizza felt there was little more planning that could be done until the hospital expressed its commitment. She and Patterson drew up a list of members of a possible hospice advisory committee, including both hospital staff and community people. Hospital officials requested its limitation to hospital personnel.

While thus attempting slowly to aggregate the support of leading officials of the hospital, Ravizza began spending more time with terminally ill patients at Strong Memorial and with *Make Today Count,* a group that works with dying people and victims of cancer. Her interviews with patients had begun when she was delineating the need for a hospice in Rochester in the feasibility study. Now she began to see more patients, and her involvement increased her friction with some hospital personnel. When Patterson asked Ravizza to talk to one of his patients, a 29-year-old man with a limited prognosis, and his wife, who was extremely upset, Ravizza began visiting them in their home and talking with them at great length. As soon as he was admitted to the hospital, hospital social workers began insinuating that she had no right to see patients. One of the oncology nurses, who became upset that Ravizza was seeing a cancer patient in the hospital, called a meeting of hospital officials and demanded that Ravizza get clearance from her before seeing any patients. Patterson supported Ravizza and reiterated that he had asked Ravizza to become involved with his patient. Once again, however, the issues of specialization and quality care were being raised. The oncology nurse did not want interference with her patients, yet she admitted that no one from the hospital intended to become supportive of this man's wife and two young children after he died.

At a meeting on November 18th, the tentative hospice advisory committee agreed to commit the hospital to becoming more involved in the creation of the hospice. The committee agreed to meet monthly to keep abreast of developments. Ravizza thought she might have a green light to develop a hospice unit at Strong, but she sensed some hesitation from officials at the meeting. Their commitment was somewhat ambiguous, certainly tentative, but no one at the meeting made any statement that might reveal why this was so.

Many details of the future hospice operation remained to be worked out. Decisions had to be made about the number of beds to be involved. A staffing ratio had to be determined and defended. A wing had to be redesigned.

A larger problem was working out the relationship of the hospice to the home care agencies. The Home Care Association is the umbrella for the Visiting Nurses and the Public Health Nurses in the area, and they make up the only voluntary, nonprofit home care-givers. The hospice would deal only with the voluntary organizations because insurance companies will pay for care by the Home Care Association agencies, but not for care from private companies.

The relationship between the home care nurses and the hospice might be complex. Negotiations by all parties would have to determine how long nurses would be able to continue seeing patients at home. A member of the hospice staff would coordinate care with the home care agencies and would go into the homes to make sure things were running smoothly and that satisfactory care was being given.

Funds were needed, since the hospital might not be willing to pay for the high staff ratio. Planning and training money as well as operating money had to be obtained so that visiting nurses, volunteers, and staff could be trained for the job. The Van Amerigen Foundation was a possible source for planning money, as was the Monroe County Cancer and Leukemia Association with which the Cancer Center enjoyed excellent relations. But two additional problems remained: finding departments willing to give up beds for the unit, and working out reimbursement by insurance companies.

There were 10 to 15 clinical chiefs in the hospital who could free beds. If they each released one bed, Ravizza reasoned, she would have the initial 12-bed unit she had decided on. Clearly, some might be more willing to release beds than others. Since there would be no pediatric patients, the pediatrics department could not be counted upon, while the medical chief might be willing to release several beds.

Dr. Bartlett, the medical director of the hospital, preferred applying to the Planning Council for the beds, but the Planning Council had already told Ravizza that they would never approve more beds because of the surplus beds in Monroe County hospitals. The petition process for more beds is at least a three-month process that would delay the opening of a hospice unit.

The other big problem, in Ravizza's view, was the question of payments from insurance. On the one hand, hospice patients would already be hospital patients and the hospice program could just be presented as another form of hospital care. However, the Executive Director of Rochester Blue Cross/Blue Shield was unwilling to commit himself, reasoning that costs could be kept down if more people died at home, even though hospice experience elsewhere strongly suggests that hospice costs are significantly lower than hospital costs.

Ravizza intended to receive help from the Genesee Region Health Planning Council and the hospital administration to work out the technical and budgetary elements of the planning. This new stage in the hospice's development was one for which Ravizza had little experience, but which she had confidence that she could handle with extra help. She reported that she needed a health planner, but it was unclear whether or not the commitment from the hospital was strong enough to fund another person.

The End of Hospice Planning at Strong

Suddenly, as a matter of great surprise to Ravizza, Dr. Patterson told her in February 1977, that the grant from which she had been paid had run out and that she would be terminated with two weeks' notice. No other explanation was given. While several compensatory gestures were made by Patterson (including paying her to attend an upcoming conference of hospice planners), and while he expressed great personal regret about the decision to dismiss her, Ravizza could not discover other reasons why she was being forced to leave and why the hospice concept was (at least temporarily) moribund at Strong Hospital.[20]

It seems likely that several reasons led to the sudden dismissal of Claire Ravizza and the demise of the hospice-within-a-hospital concept at Strong Memorial. First, and perhaps most important, support within the hospital had always been "soft." While a number of hospital officials had voiced their support, the near unanimity of opinion that might be required was lacking. The hospice advisory committee was almost an afterthought, formed *after* all the initial surveys and needs assessment had been completed. Major hospital decision makers, including important department heads, had been left out of the early planning process. A number of major figures heard of the hospice when demands were placed on them to relinquish precious beds. Many hospital personnel simply had not been sold on the desirability of a hospice before they were asked to contribute to it.

Second, the hospice planning had finally reached a stage when large-scale hospital resources would have to be committed to it. Beds, space, and personnel are far more difficult to obtain in a hospital than a salary for a single planner in an ancillary project. Coupled with the "soft" commitment, these important resources may have been impossible to obtain.

Third, outside relationships (as with home care agencies) had not been finalized.

Fourth, the all-important matter of third-party (insurance) reimbursement had not been resolved. Without that issue being decided in favor of the projected hospice, there was no point in continuing the planning or developmental process.

Fifth, the skills required by Ravizza to assess the patients' needs and initial planning and organizing were not the skills needed to effect the more technical facility-planning work, the organizing and training of staff, and the development of financial management procedures. Indeed, as Claire Ravizza herself recognized, organizing support for a hospice concept is very different from preparing to make one operationally sound. The hospital was not prepared to hire additional staff for such planning when the other unresolved issues remained.

Sixth, some physicians, including a few important department chiefs, simply refused to give up beds to a new unit. They resented anyone who made such a request.

And seventh, Ravizza herself may have incurred some lasting resentment among a few people when she used some spare time to try to give support to a few dying patients.

Most of these objections could have been resolved. But the dying do not speak loudly and they have no lobby, certainly not within a large medical establishment like Strong Memorial Hospital.

8

The Hospice Movement

The hospice "movement," as it may be called, has planning groups in virtually every major, and many smaller, cities across the United States. These organizations are at many different stages of development, ranging from discussion groups of interested citizens, through functional planning organizations involving health care professionals, to operating groups with facilities actually offering hospice services, usually on an outpatient basis but often with an inpatient facility on the drawing boards.

It is not yet clear what population level is necessary to sustain an inpatient hospice facility, but it would appear from the planning by the Strong Memorial Hospital group in Rochester that an urban population of approximately 300,000, or a combined urban and suburban population of 750,000 will supply considerably more than the critical mass of dying people required to support a hospice care unit. While it is known how many people are likely to die in a given population, and from what causes (see Chap. 2), the proportion willing to use different types of hospice services is not yet known. By late 1978, however, there were planning groups committed to the development of hospice care programs in no fewer than 115 cities across the United States.[1]

Hospice of Santa Barbara, Inc. in California has sponsored lengthy public education programs in a three-county area, and has trained volunteers and professionals to participate in a home care program. The full range of community-based professional personnel from physicians to social workers are being trained to deal with issues of death and dying in a series of workshops and seminars. While Hospice of Santa Barbara, Inc. does not as yet provide direct services to patients or their families, a sensitive information referral service is offered which maintains contact with existing human service agencies and specific personnel who have received special training to handle problems of death.

Hospice of Buffalo, New York, with local funding for two years of planning operations, has supported conferences on the care of the dying and is gauging the support in the community while constantly gathering key medical personnel to its cause. Its activities indicate some of the principal concerns of most other hospice efforts: obtaining support among physicians, developing community support, obtaining local financing, approaching the National Cancer Institute for federal-level support, involving health care agencies (e.g., visiting nurses' services), training professionals from other agencies, affiliating (or not affiliating) with one or more hospitals, and working for reimbursement from public and private insurance programs.

Two hospitals in New York City provide delivery of hospice-type care within a hospital setting: Calvary Hospital in the Bronx and St. Luke's in Manhattan.

CALVARY HOSPITAL

One-third of all deaths from cancer in New York City occur in Calvary Hospital, which is classified as a chronic disease hospital. Patients are admitted with a minimum of three weeks of life remaining and a maximum of approximately six weeks. Because of the purposes of Calvary Hospital, they average as many as one or two deaths each day. Ninety-two hospitals in the region refer patients to Calvary, often when these patients are known to be approaching death. Daily care at Calvary costs exactly half that of a well-known acute care hospital for cancer patients nearby, but is approximately the same costs as some other, less renowned nearby hospitals that do not focus on dying patients.

Hospice-type features at Calvary include: the assignment of one primary physician to each patient, the establishment of two constant care units with 24 beds for patients who need to receive continual surveillance, a well-organized recreation program that includes trips for patients to nearby special events such as operas and plays, and the provision of day rooms for patient use.

On the other hand, Calvary lacks some other features of a typical hospice program. There has never been a home care service at Calvary, although the need for one is recognized. There is no treatment of bereaving family members. Calvary's primary emphasis is on proper medical management of the cancer patient, an important function in a society that often fails to provide even good medical care to such patients. However, Calvary still remains very much a hospital, with restricted access to entrances and floors and with the traditional hospital physical environment of long corridors and one community meeting room per floor. Although the medical needs of the patients are attended to scrupulously, no effort is made to deal with the psychological or emotional problems of patients. Family members do not receive any special supportive services although visiting hours are extended as death approaches.

St. Luke's Hospital

Many more hospice-type features can be found at St. Luke's Hospital in Manhattan. The hospice program at St. Luke's began in 1975 with a special hospice team that works with five to ten patients scattered throughout the hospital. The primary objective of the hospice project at St. Luke's is the comfort of patients and their families with a view towards what staff term "constructive living." Patients are informed that they are hospice patients, although a patient does not necessarily have to know his prognosis in order to be a designated patient. These patients receive special privileges and extra attention from hospice staff, which consists of a coordinator, two half-time nurses, half-time physician, a half-time social worker, and additional voluntary assistance from chaplains and others. The patient's physician and family must indicate their willingness to participate, and the patient must give evidence of an advanced stage of cancer. Preference is given to patients whose symptoms are not being controlled.

The special privileges include extra visitors outside normal visiting hours. Children, and even occasionally a pet, are allowed to visit, and an apartment is available in the nurses' residence to enable visitors to stay overnight. Patients are allowed alcoholic beverages at intervals determined by the primary physician.

In addition, approximately ten outpatients receive care from the hospice team. The coordinator and the social workers visit these patients at home and the hospice provides emergency assistance for patients with special needs. A volunteer program is being developed to help patients travel and feed themselves, and to bring medication to these home-bound patients.

The hospice team recognizes that it has little contact with families to date. They do not provide around-the-clock service; there have been no research projects, inservice education, or moral-boosting staff sessions, which are all parts of a well-developed hospice program.

There are clearly some advantages to the St. Luke's project. The regular staff on the floors throughout the hospital can observe first-hand the care that should be given to terminal patients. The St. Luke's model may be the only alternative available to some hospitals and small communities with severely limited space and resources and therefore unable to set aside a special unit or facility for terminal care. Furthermore, whatever stigma may attach to a special unit for dying patients may be avoided.

In contrast to these advantages, however, are several obvious disadvantages of the St. Luke's model. Because hospice patients are singled out for special privileges, there may be repercussions and resentment from other patients or family members. Furthermore, it is clearly very difficult to develop a supportive atmosphere for terminally ill patients when they are scattered throughout the hospital. As in the care with Calvary Hospital, the severe limitations imposed by the traditional hospital's physical environment may be altered.

OTHER HOSPICES

Hospice of Marin, Inc., of Kentfield, California has a volunteer staff consisting of registered nurses, Masters of Social Work, a physician, and family counselors. A small home care program is in operation, and an inpatient service is being planned. The group consults with primary care physicians (especially as regards pain management) and provides important psychological services to patients, families, nursing services and clergy.

Hospice Atlanta, in Georgia, functions as a program of the Unitarian congregation. They are planning a day-care center for the incurably ill, a home care program, and a licensed, skilled nursing facility.

Hospices are being developed in many different ways, some of which differ slightly from the basic models presented in earlier chapters. For example, some hospices are being planned with very large numbers of voluntary, community-based planners; with small numbers of highly trained, professional volunteers who are actually providing medical services; as part of church-based efforts to respond to the needs of the dying; as part of nursing home operations; and with novel concepts such as a day-care program for the terminally ill. Cities now providing hospice services or supporting hospice planners are listed in the footnotes to this chapter.

While some of these planners and planning groups are not likely to get past the early talking stages, others have most of the necessary resources already at their disposal. Many cities have more than one hospice planning organization, and a few have as many as four such groups.

The entire group of hospice planning organizations across the nation deserves the term "movement." It is slowly, rationally, and carefully planning the development of a national network of terminal care facilities. Some will fail, certainly, but many will succeed. The entire network deserves the attention of lay people and health care specialists alike. For better or worse, these planners, usually highly committed and well-situated within their local communities, are likely to affect the quality of dying all Americans experience.

9

The Federal Response

Partly because the most likely candidates for modern hospice care are cancer patients, and partly because the federal government has no other agency or mechanism with which to fund hospices, the federal response to the hospice movement has been directed through the National Cancer Institute. The National Cancer Institute (NCI) in Bethesda, Maryland is the federal government's principal agency for research on cancer prevention, diagnosis, treatment, and rehabilitation, and for dissemination of information on the control of cancer. The NCI was established by the National Cancer Act of 1937 as part of the Public Health Service. It is one of 11 institutes and 4 divisions that make up the National Institutes of Health of the Department of Health, Education and Welfare.

The National Cancer Act of 1971 directed the Institute to "plan and develop an expanded, intensified, and coordinated cancer research program encompassing the program of the National Cancer Institute, related programs of the other research institutes, and other Federal and non-

Federal programs."[1] To speed the translation of research results into widespread application, the act authorized a cancer control program to demonstrate and communicate to both the medical community and the general public the latest advances in cancer prevention and management.

The act directed the establishment of a network of comprehensive cancer centers located around the country. These centers engage in a wide range of cancer-related activities, encompassing basic research, diagnosis, treatment, and rehabilitation, and professional education and training in the various clinical and research disciplines. The centers attempt to stimulate cancer care throughout the nation through demonstration and outreach programs.

The legislation also established a three-member President's Cancer Panel appointed by the President of the United States to monitor development and execution of the National Cancer Program. At least two members of the panel are scientists or physicians appointed for three-year terms. In addition, the National Cancer Advisory Board of 23 members (18 non-federal-government experts appointed by the President and 5 government officials as ex-officio members) advises the Director of NCI on the National Cancer Program.

The National Cancer Act Amendments of 1974 extended the National Cancer program for three years, and amended the authorities to provide a larger national program, including the establishment of additional Comprehensive Cancer Centers.

Research supported by the Institute is organized into the broad areas of cancer biology, cause and prevention, detection and diagnosis, treatment, and rehabilitation. This spectrum of research is conducted through five divisions: Cancer Cause and Prevention, Cancer Biology and Diagnosis, Cancer Treatment, Cancer Research Resources and Centers, and Cancer Control and Rehabilitation. The Institute's intramural research is conducted in laboratories in Bethesda, Maryland, and at the NIH Clinical Center,

Bethesda; at the Veterans Administration Hospital in Washington, D.C.; the Baltimore Cancer Research Center in Baltimore, Maryland; and at the Frederick Cancer Research Center, Ft. Detrick, Maryland.

Research in cancer biology explores the basic processes of life and malignant changes. The cancer biology program focuses on the transformation of normal cells into cancerous ones and on factors affecting the growth of cancer cells. The research also includes basic laboratory studies of the process by which possible carcinogenic agents, such as viruses, interact with cell components to cause cell transformation. Related studies are concerned with the alteration of that process to prevent cancer.

The program for prevention of cancer and identification of its causes covers the following broad areas; epidemiologic studies to identify population groups in whom cancer occurs more, or less, frequently than in the general population (thus providing clues to causative factors); studies of chemical and physical agents that may cause cancer; studies of viruses as a possible cause of cancer; and studies of the cancer-causing process (carcinogenesis).

The primary goal of research in cancer detection is to develop the means for detecting cancer when the disease is in its early stages and thus more amenable to cure. Research is also directed toward the development of techniques for screening large numbers of people.

The long-term objective of cancer treatment is to cure or effectively control cancer in humans. Scientists and physicians are working to increase the number of patients responding to therapy and to prolong the period of disease-free remission and survival. The National Cancer Program emphasizes the development of combinations of treatment methods for each type of cancer. New drugs are being studied in combination with other drugs and with surgery and irradiation.

Rehabilitation programs of the Institute are conducted by the Division of Cancer Control and Rehabilitation. Research and demonstration projects deal with facets of the rehabilitation of the cancer patient, from palliative and restorative aspects to problems of a vocational or psychological nature. In keeping with the concept of the "comprehensive" cancer center, the institute supports efforts in developing and demonstrating rehabilitative services for patients within the framework of multidisciplinary centers.

When Congress authorized the establishment of the National Cancer Institute in 1937, with all of the then 96 senators supporting the bill, the stage was set for most of the biomedical research in cancer and other diseases through the postwar period. Fellowship programs, research, grants, antinarcotic programs, and the construction of hospitals and research facilities all proceeded as the following additional national institutes were established in 1948 to 1950: The National Heart Institute; the National Institute of Dental Research; the National Microbiological Institute; the National Institute of Mental Health; the National Institute of Arthritis and Metabolic Diseases; and the National Institute of Neurological Diseases and Blindness.

In 1953 the Public Health Service became part of the newly created Department of Health, Education and Welfare and the rest of the 1950s and all of the 1960s saw the proliferation of research projects; various types of training programs, divisions, subdivisions, and centers for specific health-related problems; enabling acts to obtain ever-broader powers; survey programs; research facilities; libraries; and international projects. This has all resulted in the national institutes and eight special support centers, divisions, and libraries.

The astronomical growth in the size of the National Institutes of Health is best indicated by their budgets. From $464,000 in total appropriations for 1938, the national institutes grew to spend $430,000,000 in 1960 and an astounding $2,089,897,000 in 1975. The National Cancer Institute has always retained the largest share of the budget.

If these appropriations are broken down by functional area, the National Cancer Institute has nearly always spent more money for research grants than the other institutes of health, and it rivals the National Heart and Lung Institute and the National Institute of Arthritis, Metabolism, and Digestive Diseases in money spent for training grants and fellowships.

The National Cancer Institute justifies these expenditures by pointing to the shear bulk of its contracts for research relating to the cause, prevention, detection, diagnosis, and treatment of cancer, and its therapy and rehabilitation programs. NCI makes grants to universities, hospitals, laboratories, and other public and private nonprofit institutions for research. It supports professional education in cancer research, including clinical cancer research, through individual research fellowships and project grants.

In late 1971 and early 1972, NCI convened a series of 40 meetings by 250 nonfederal and federal scientists to assist in the development of the National Cancer Program Plan which consists of two major documents: The Strategic Plan, which presents a series of recommendations for cancer research and cancer control activities; and the National Cancer Program Operational Plan, which describes the National Cancer Program operations and the major policies and procedures for management and operation of the National Cancer Program. It also outlines the major directions the National Cancer Program will pursue for the next five years.

The National Advisory Cancer Council is a body of appointed members and ex-officio members created by law to advise on general policies and needs, and to review the status of research and the application of research results in fields pertinent to cancer. The members of the council are appointed to staggered terms of 4 years each. The Director of the National Institutes of Health, or his or her representative serves as Chairperson of the Council, ex-officio. The other two ex-officio members are a medical officer designated by the Secretary of Defense and the chief medical officer of the Veteran's Administration or his or her representative. Of the appointive members, not less than half are required to be scientists or physicians skilled and experienced in the problems of cancer. Other members may be from educational and research fields or be public-spirited citizens interested in the cancer problem. In addition to general policy and program recommendations, the council reviews and recommends appropriate action on applications for grants-in-aid for research and for training related to cancer.[2]

The National Cancer Institute Director has responsibility for a seven-month planning period in which the central administration and the NCI divisions update goals, prepare proposals based on that revised goal setting, state priorities for new programs, and send the completed proposal for review and "sign off" to the National Cancer Advisory Board. A five-month period of formalizing the proposal follows. During this crucial period the proposal is mainly out of the hands of the NCI Director, as the National Institutes of Health and the staff of Department of the Health, Education and Welfare review and comment on it before sending it to the Office of Management and Budget (OMB) and the White House, which together prepare the President's Budget Message to Congress. OMB and the President's staff are concerned almost entirely not with the three stages of goal setting, planning, and programming, but with the budget review process. By this time, these four reviews have consumed a full year. When the President's budget is transmitted to Congress, an additional six months is spent preparing guidelines and justifications for the Congress, going through Congressional appropriations hearings, and having the final Appropriations Bill passed and signed into law. The major responsibility for substantive, nonfinancial aspects of National Cancer Institute policies is held by the NCI Director and staff, with review and comment provided by the Advisory Board. The National Institutes of Health, and the Secretary of HEW, OMB and the Office of the President are concerned primarily with budgetary matters, although they always have the option of intruding substantive concerns into their review process. The appropriate Congressional staffs (primarily of health committees in both Houses of Congress) may, if they wish, link substantive planning concerns with budgetary concerns. But such a linkage rarely concerns the congressional staff when considering such a relatively sacred matter as a cancer control plan backed by the entire established medical profession as represented by NCI and the other national institutes. Congress always seems to have other, more pressing concerns.

Some idea of the substantive priorities of NCI, however, may easily be determined by examining closely the annual budget. A breakdown of the NCI fiscal year 1974 budget is shown in Table 1.[3]

Grant-supported programs of the NCI are administered chiefly by the Division of Cancer Research Resources and

Table 1
NCI Budget for Fiscal Year 1974.

	Amount ($)	Percent of Total
Research contracts	94,964,000	16.3
Research support contracts	72,365,000	12.5
Research grants	198,960,000	34.2
Research support grants	44,345,000	7.6
Total construction costs	38,090,000	6.6
Total management costs	45,786,000	7.9
In-house research	31,289,000	5.4
In-house "support"	9,040,000	1.6
Interagency agreements	15,114,000	2.6
Cancer control	31,161,000	5.3

Source: Adapted from *National Cancer Institute fact book*, p. 25.

Centers.[4] The activities of the grant-supported program are in the areas of prevention, detection, causes, and treatment of the many forms of cancer and rehabilitation of the cancer patient, as well as basic research. NCI awards grants for basic research studies; clinical studies; cancer centers; construction and renovation of research facilities; personnel development, training, and education; and cancer control.

Under procedures approved by the Director of the National Institutes of Health, the Direcror of NCI may approve grants in amounts less than $35,000. Grant requests exceeding $35,000 must be approved by the National Cancer Advisory Board. The board receives advice on grant applications from peer review committees of scientists recognized as authorities in the various health science disciplines. For each proposal, a critical assessment is made of the scientific merit of the project, the ability of the investigator, the adequacy of available facilities, and the overall significance of the project.

The services of profit-making organizations are extensively utilized in the National Cancer Program through the contract mechanism. Contracts for specific projects are solicited through requests for proposals that are advertised in the *Commerce Business Daily,* a publication of the U.S. Department of Commerce. Directions for submitting proposals are contained in these notices. Organizations wishing to suggest contract projects not specifically requested by NCI may submit unsolicited proposals, but these appear to receive a lower priority for funding. Contract proposals are reviewed by Technical Review Committees of scientific peers in much the same way as grant proposals. It is obvious that most of the people who make decisions on either grant or contract proposals are well established, respected professionals.

In addition to looking at an NCI budget by functional areas, another way of breaking down the NCI budget is to organize it into NCI divisions. Table 2 does this for the 1975 budget (amounts are in thousands of dollars).[5]

Table 2
1975 NCI Budget

Activity	Amount ($)	Percent of Total
Division of Cancer Research Resources and Centers		
Regular Program	135,515	19.6
Cancer research centers	115,834	16.7
Task forces (organ sites)	12,000	1.8
Research career program	2,000	0.3
Radiation development	4,250	0.6
Clinical education program	5,000	0.7
Fellowships	12,066	1.7
Training grants	10,097	1.5
Construction	30,000	4.3
Review and approval	6,222	0.9
Total	332,984	48.1
Division of Cancer Biology and Diagnosis		
Laboratory and clinical research	41,711	6.0
Task forces	9,085	1.3
Total	50,796	7.3
Division of Cancer Treatment		
Cancer therapy	82,125	11.9
Task forces	750	0.1
Total	82,875	12.0
Division of Cancer Cause and Prevention		
Office of division director	11,171	1.6
Virus cancer program	57,884	8.4
Carcinogenesis	35,794	5.2
Field studies and statistics	11,924	1.7
Task forces	5,580	0.8
Total	122,353	17.7
Division of Cancer Control and Rehabilitation		
Cancer control	50,098	7.3

(Continued)

Table 2   (Continued)

Activity	Amount ($)	Percent of Total
Office of the director		
Program direction and supporting services	25,412	3.7
Management fund	19,148	2.7
Construction contracts	8,000	1.2
Total	52,560	7.6
TOTAL	$691,666	100.0

Source: NIH 76-792, p. 27.
Table 3 shows the same 1975 budget broken down into large program areas.[6]

Table 3 shows the same 1975 budget broken down into large program areas.[6]

These tables have been presented in order to demonstrate one of the primary problems facing a service-oriented movement such as the hospice movement: the national priorities present very few opportunities for organizations concerned with cancer victims, those whom the national cancer program fails in one sense, to make demands on the national purse. Only the cancer control portion of the national budget—a relatively miniscule portion indeed—can be allocated to services delivered to terminal victims of cancer. In fact, cancer control funds were first appropriated as separate budget items only in 1973.[7] Of course, the Cancer Control portion of the NCI budget is not entirely available to groups delivering services to cancer patients. In Table 4, the budgetary obligations for cancer control for 1974 and 1975 are presented.[8]

The claims made by hospice groups, of course, may be placed against the last category only, which is slightly more than half of the cancer control budget, which in turn amounts to only 7.4% of the total NCI budget. It is interest-

Table 3
1975 Budget by Program Areas

	Amount ($)	Percent of Total
Research	547,200,000	79.1
Construction, planning, support of centers, and manpower development	93,366,000	13.5
Cancer control	51,100,000	7.4

Source: NIH 76-792, p. 28.

Table 4
Budget for Cancer Control.

	Total 1974 ($)	1974 (%)	Total 1975 ($)	1975 (%)
Detection, diagnosis, pre-treatment evaluation	10,438,000	30.9	17,898,000	35.7
Prevention	3,792,000	11.2	4,899,000	9.8
Treatment, rehabilitation, continuing care	19,527,000	57.9	27,302,000	54.5

Source: NIH 76-792, p. 30.

ing to note from the figures that while the total dollars allocated for treatment and continuing care have risen considerably in the 1974 and 1975 fiscal years, the proportions of the total NCI budget, and the cancer control sub-budget, given over to this category began to decline, and have continued to decline since then.

Activities of the Cancer Control Program involve community hospitals, state and local health departments, and lay and voluntary organizations in a wide variety of cancer care programs. In 1975, $4,400,000 were spent in cancer control grants, $43,998,000 in various types of cancer control contracts, and $1,700,000 in administrative and other in-house costs.[9]

The Cancer Control Programs fall under three titles: prevention; detection, diagnosis, and pretreatment evaluation; and treatment, rehabilitation, and continuing care.[10] Hospices fall into the last category.

Prevention is concerned with the dissemination of information to the public and to health professionals regarding techniques and methods to halt the spread of cancer.[11] The program promotes an understanding of industrial carcinogens and other environmental hazards, along with motivational methods to establish positive attitudes and practices among professional, labor, and management groups. The total budget for all programs associated with prevention was $2.9 million in 1974 to a projected $36 million in 1980. The drastic increase in this budget from 1974 to 1980 largely represents personnel costs. Where NCI had 225 scientists working in this area in 1974, it expects to have 2,153 working in 1980.

Detection, diagnosis, and pretreatment evaluation is concerned with the continuous assessment and widespread utilization of modern detection methods. New cancer-screening techniques are evaluated and demonstrated. The program tries to promote the most efficient use of facilities and personnel, and education to improve professional levels of performance in the vital area of detection. From a budget of $14 million in 1974, the total program budget is expected to rise to $61 million in 1980. The largest portions of these yearly budgets go to screening and detection methods. As in the prevention program, the dramatic increases in the detection, diagnosis, and pretreatment evaluation program's yearly budget for 1974 to 1980 is accounted for by a very large increase in the number of scientists NCI expects to have working in this area, from 1,101 in 1974 to 3,646 in 1980.

The treatment, rehabilitation, and continuing care program tries to assure that optimal treatment, rehabilitation, and palliative care methods are available to cancer patients. The program is concerned with disseminating information regarding new treatments, methods to improve professional and public acceptance of the new methods, and techniques for community home care and other types of care (including hospices). The budget for treatment, rehabilitation, and continuing care will rise from $15 million in 1974 to $97 million in 1980. As with the other two cancer control programs, the greatest increases over the period are in the area of personnel. The number of NCI-supported physicians expected to be working on this program will rise from 1,449 in 1974 to 5,922 in 1980. The greatest portion of the program's budget goes to the assessment of treatment and follow-up methods. As much smaller portion goes to rehabilitation methods, while relatively very little is allocated to palliative and supportive care methods. In millions of dollars, Table 5 provides a comparison of palliative and supportive care allocations to total treatment, rehabilitation, and continuing care allocation. It appears likely that money for *all* palliative measures will represent a decreasing portion of the overall budget.

What does this review of NCI's structure and functions tell us about the likelihood that the federal government will respond positively to increasing demands from hospice planners? Some pessimism regarding a positive response seems warranted, and the following 22 conclusions drawn from the above review of NCI operations support that pessimism.

Table 5
Comparison of Allocations in Millions of Dollars[11]

	Palliative and Supportive Care	Treatment, Rehabilitation Continuing Care Total
1974	0.914	14.702
1975	1.370	19.746
1976	2.322	30.400
1980 (projected)	10.000	97.000

1. The network of comprehensive cancer centers located around the country does not coincide with the developing network of groups interested in hospices. Many hospice groups exist in areas not served directly by the high-powered, highly financed cancer centers. Strong's planned hospice clearly was aided by its relationship to the Strong Cancer Center—in terms of the easy availability of patients, the support of oncologists and other professionals, and access to money—but many hospice planning groups are not so fortunate.

2. The President's Cancer Panel, which monitors the National Cancer Program and is required to have at least two-thirds of its members composed of scientists and physicians, and the National Cancer Advisory Board, which oversees NCI's operation of the National Cancer Program and has about 75 percent of its membership composed of well-recognized, Presidentially-appointed "professionals," are not likely to be the strongest representatives of consumer (cancer patients') interests. Indeed, the people appointed to both the panel and the board are successful practitioners of the present war on cancer. They have enjoyed a professional lifetime of interest in the way that war is conducted. The failures of their system, the terminal cancer victims, are more easily ignored than held up to the public spotlight.

   a. The professional orientation of the generals in the war on cancer is to continue the way that war is conducted; indeed, they know no other way.

   b. The very recruitment of those generals, on the basis of prestige within the professions, suggests a conservative continuation of current strategies.

   c. The recruitment of the generals of the war on cancer is almost entirely from provider groups, not people who have cancer or who expect to get it. That fact alone may suggest both that cancer victims will not receive much sympathy in the allocations the physician-scientist-generals make, and that more emphasis will be placed on prevention and detection than on palliative care for the victims. This is not necessarily to suggest that the priorities are immoral, only that they may be both self-serving and unsympathetic to competing demands from cancer victims.

    d. There is virtually no consumer interest group representation in the recruitment process that selects the generals in the war on cancer. No group aggregates or articulates consumer interests in the selection of the leaders of war.

    e. The practices that the leaders in the war on cancer have engaged in are associated with aggressive therapy. Their professional orientation to their patients is vigorously curative in nature, not palliative.

3. The entire history of the National Institute of Health, from the 1878 Federal Quarantine Act "for investigating the origin and causes of epidemic diseases" to the present, has been focused on etiological research, and not nearly as much as on palliative care. Hospice planners fly in the face of a long-established tradition, actually a cultural orientation, which states that prevention is better than cure and which consequently tends to downplay some cures, and certainly writes off those patients who have no hope of cure. This cure orientation may be seriously inappropriate now that major causes of death are reduced to a handful of diseases for which there is little information after the expenditure of billions of dollars, dozens of years, and millions of lives.

4. The tradition of federal efforts in the health field also emphasizes laboratory work and lab results to find

better ways of providing care to victims. Research facilities have always received a heavy emphasis when compared to facilities that provide care.

5. Training funds provided by the National Cancer Institute are spent for programs that perpetuate the aggressive therapy, cure-provider orientations of the related professions.

6. Education funds also continue the tradition of emphasizing cure over care. We do not like to look at the victims, so we emphasize instead those hopeful statements that suggest the rest of us have a decreasing likelihood of catching the disease.

7. Contract programs continue the traditions and emphasis of the grant programs, especially because contracts are usually awarded to established (and therefore long-recognized members of the medical "establishment") organizations, as well as to private research labs.

8. The National Cancer Program's Strategic Plan and Operational Plan were devised by 250 scientists and physicians who were providers of research, not providers of care, and certainly not consumers of care. They continue the programs, policies, and procedures for the operation of the National Cancer Program that has been described here as not very conducive to hospice planning groups.

9. The structure of the NCI is designed to stress certain responsibilities that are not favorable to allocation requests from hospice organizations. None of the associate directors under the director, nor the assistant and deputy directors has any responsibility for the palliative care of the victims of the war they are waging. Only two of the five directors of major divisions might have any such concern.

10. An examination of job descriptions and structural charts suggests strongly that neither of the two division directors who may have a concern for palliative

care modalities is likely to emphasize that concern. The director for cancer treatment has associate directors for aggressive therapy evaluation, medical oncology, experimental therapeutics for people who may "recover," and for the Baltimore Center, which concentrates on laboratory and clinical research. The director of cancer control and rehabilitation is primarily concerned with prevention, the evaluation of detection and diagnosis programs, and communications. A very small portion of his or her total function is concerned with continuing care, and this includes (and emphasizes) treatment and rehabilitation rather than terminal care.

11. The NCI proportions of the total resources committed to the entire national war on cancer amount to 65 percent of all money spent on the war each year. Other federal agencies spend 9 percent, while state and local governments contribute an additional 9 percent. Thus slightly more than 83 percent of all money spent on cancer-related operations and programs in this nation is public money, and virtually all of it is heavily influenced by federal priorities. The rest of cancer funding (from voluntary agencies, private institutions, and industry) is also heavily influenced by the preponderant, even overwhelming, position of the NCI and its funding priorities.

12. The budget development and administration process is not conducive to applications from hospice planning groups, for at least these three reasons:

   a. The budget justification procedures are heavily oriented toward established institutions with "track records." New groups find it very difficult to break into the total set of justifications for the huge NCI budget because they have no successful experience on which to base their claims.

   b. The 18-month budget process is so long that it favors established institutions that expect minimal deviations (nearly always increases) in their usual financial requirements. The accurate projections of a budget for a brand new institution 18 months in advance is extremely difficult because of the complex network of independent factors that affect costs and cannot be predicted with certainty without some financial experience extending over several years.

    c. The budget review process has no important access for new program justifications. Only the relatively short Congressional review portion of the entire process offers any possibility of a structured means to articulate the need for a new project and insert it into the budget. Yet the Congressional hearings stage has never yet resulted in any substantial change in the budgets and justifications submitted by the Executive Branch to the Congress. This may be because health and cancer-related programs are usually "sacred cows," with strong, wealthy, organized support from vested interests, with little consumer participation, and little organized opposition on complex issue and culturally distasteful subjects.

13. Substantive priorities are implied by budgeting allocations, and the breakdowns of the NCI budget presented earlier suggests again that palliative care is an extremely small part of the NCI priorities.

14. Grants and contracts are awarded for different reasons, but both seem strongly oriented towards the established policies that make it difficult for hospice groups to obtain a fair hearing.

15. Some of the principal criteria used to award grants are difficult for consumer-oriented hospice planning groups to meet. The "scientific merit" of a hospice project may be considered minimal. The "ability of the investigator" may not be relevant, and most hos-

pices tend to downplay interruptive research. The "significance of the project in relation to the need for knowledge" may be similarly minimal.

16. Contracts with profit-making organizations are usually awarded for small, well-delineated services or products, not for general, overall care programs. NCI has very little experience in contracting for or evaluating overall treatment programs.

17. The NCI budget when broken down into divisions again suggests strongly the low priority attached to palliative care. The same is true when the budget's large program areas are examined. Indeed, only half the cancer control budget, which in turn is only 7.4 percent of the total NCI budget, is available for cancer control programs that *may* include hospice claims. Unfortunately, the relative position of this part of the NCI budget is declining.

18. In the NCI planning structure there is no direct responsibility for palliative care planning functions.

19. Both the job security and longevity associated with administrative and planning jobs in NCI, on the one hand, and the professional training available to the newer NCI recruits, on the other, suggests that the professional orientations of NCI personnel are not likely to change quickly from a more traditional, conservative approach to one that is open to palliative care programs.

20. NCI planners describe their jobs as developing new program plans by working with existing programs and operating program personnel. The influences they acknowledge are not conducive to the development of alternative institutions.

21. The Formulation Branch of the staff is concerned with etiology, prevention, and diagnosis. The Planning Branch, too, is concerned with operations planning techniques and biomedical research. These

           functions are strongly supportive of existing institutional arrangements, to the virtual exclusion of alternative structures.

22. NCI's largest budgetary resources have been, and are projected to be, in the employment of natural scientists—not social scientists, policy analysts, evaluators, planners, or public health specialists. These latter groups of professionals, of course, are needed to participate in the sound development of a hospice network.

In short, from every vantage point the NCI response to the hospice movement—structural organization, job descriptions of key personnel, functional analysis, budgetary allocations suggestive of priorities, the nature of the NCI budgetary process itself, the training and types of personnel available to the organization, the objectives of the substantive programs NCI operates, its history and traditions, and the backgrounds and attitudes of the men who oversee and direct the organization—it is a reasonable conclusion that NCI is not prepared to engage in the proper goal setting, planning, programming, development and allocation of resources, and evaluation processes that are required for a positive, well-coordinated federal approach to the hospice movement.

Even with all of these obstacles to a positive and effective NCI response to the hospice movement, the agency has had a response. As Lawrence Burke, formerly the NCI Program Director for Rehabilitation Treatment, told the author in 1977, "We in Cancer Control have a problem with the historic priorities. We recognized several years ago that the interchange between clinical practice and the research labs is inadequate."[12] Burke went on to say that the products of the research laboratories (usually drugs) often get transmitted easily to the physicians practicing in the field, but the experiences of the physicians and their patients are not frequently communicated to the laboratory scientists. The statement that cancer patients often suffer terribly in spite of (and sometimes because of) the chemotherapies developed by the labs rarely is made directly to the labs. Burke's conclusion is that "if our drugs make a person prey to a more ignoble death, we have even more responsibility to help them."

It was primarily for this reason that in 1974 the National Cancer Institute issued a request for proposals (RFP) that solicited suggestions and plans for the "Development and Utilization of Rehabilitation and/or Continuing Care Resources and Services."[13] In this document, NCI invited a number of groups to request funding for hospice-type programs, and, privately, NCI had decided to make up to $1 million available for the purpose.

In NCI terms, this is not a large amount of money. Still, the idea precipitated some controversy among NCI's staff, many of whom remain committed to what Burke termed the agency's "historic priorities." Burke added, "people in biomedical research resent the taking of money from those priorities, namely research." The RFP was sent out, however, because the amount of money allocated for hospices was relatively quite small. As Burke said about his later efforts with a second RFP in 1978: "They are letting me pursue this because it has been almost harmless."[14]

The 1974 request for proposals expressed an ironic rationale for hospices, in view of the reluctance of the biomedical research staff to allocate money for them: "Rehabilitation of the cancer patient has become an argument and important challenge due to the increasing number of 'cured' patients, as well as those who develop recurrent or metastic cancer, and require long range rehabilitation and/or continuing care services."[15] In other words, NCI funding priorities ought to be shifted slightly away from an exclusive focus on research because that research has been so successful that more and more survivors are demanding follow-up care. In addition, the staff might begin to think about some continuing care services to those who are not cured. For the first time among NCI programs, a small sop was thrown to the more than two-thirds of all cancer victims who are not cured.

A distinction was drawn between rehabilitation and continuing care. As the RFP stated clearly, the two terms[16]

> are not synonymous and the proposed programs should reflect a clear understanding of the distinction between the two. Rehabilitation is that process that seeks to restore optimal physical, social and vocational functioning lost as a result of injury or disease. It may be initiated prior to, during or following the major medical therapy.
>
> Continuing care, then, is that activity or endeavor which seeks to provide the required support and services needed by those cancer patients whose cancer will not be controlled or cured. Such patients following major therapy and subsequent discharge from the hospital will require a wide range of resources to ensure maximum living and death with dignity.

The "continuing care" portion of the RFP was a major breakthrough for NCI, and the importance of follow-up care to cancer patients generally was hammered home with two additional rationales: First, "radical surgery, chemotherapy and radiation therapy often leave patients with severe secondary impairments."[17] The therapies thus far developed for victims of cancer have such severe consequences that frequently patients must be helped to recover from them. And second, "It is well documented that a major crises (sic) for the cancer patient is that period immediately following discharge when the highly skilled medical care and the supportive milieu of the hospital is terminated."[18] The crisis often interferes with both the recovery of "cured" patients and the functioning of dying patients. NCI, for the first time, formally recognized that "During the post-discharge period, it is desirable to have a full spectrum of resources, hospital-based, community based and/or available at home in order to provide continuity of care for either category of oncology patients."[19]

While the RFP represented a theoretical breakthrough for NCI, it should be recognized that it was not well known or distributed. It was, in Mr. Burke's words several years later, relatively "harmless."

In fact, only Hospice, Inc. submitted a full blown proposal that met the following NCI guidelines for acceptable proposals:

Provides nursing care and visitations
Provides supportive counseling to patient and family
Provides continuing care at home
Identifies the continuing care needs of oncology patients
Identifies the resources and services needed for continuing care
Educates health care specialists
Evaluates the benefits of the program
Is cost effective
Does not overlap existing programs
Develops methods to increase "team competence," so that the program will be multidisciplinary and well-integrated
Is expertly administered
Maintains good coordination with existing, community-based services

The planning and development process for hospices explained in this book generally meet these 12 criteria. With the exception of the provision for an evaluation plan, the remaining 11 NCI requirements refer to essential components of successful hospice programs. It is instructive that NCI was requesting information (because they did not have that information but were willing to pay for it) that represents standard operating procedures in existing hospice programs and plans. These procedures and principles of good hospice care had been discovered by NCI at St. Christopher's, and the RFP explicitly admitted a reliance on the model provided by the London hospice:[20]

> The objective of this procurement is to provide a limited demonstration program to field test in the United States the St. Christopher's Hospice concept for care of the terminal cancer patient. While social/cultural differences between England and the United States may very well preclude exact duplication of all aspects of the St. Christopher's Hospice, it is requisite that the St. Christopher's philosophy of care be reflected and implemented in the offeror's proposed program.

Only Hospice, Inc. submitted a complete and acceptable proposal, and it was over 100 pages in length. The proposal and the grant they received (for nearly the $1 million NCI had available for this purpose in 1974) are described in Chapter 6.

The evaluation plan submitted by Hospice, Inc. included a detailed survey of the next of kin of cancer victims and specific measures of how well the hospice tended to the physical and nonphysical needs of patients and families. More than a year later, NCI hired an anthropologist to evaluate the Hospice, Inc. program and, first, to develop his own measures of success. When he later reported that he was too inexperienced with hospice practices to carry out an evaluation, his contract was terminated. No evaluation of the success and failures of the first NCI grant for hospice care was completed and published—another indication of the priority the agency attaches to hospice programs for dying victims of cancer.

Early in 1976, NCI officials resurrected the 1974 RFP, with its attached rationales for continuing and rehabilitative care, and decided to make another effort to test the hospice concept. A second RFP,[21] far lengthier and more detailed, was sent to cancer centers and various hospice groups and hospitals around the country. This time $3 million was made available but later reduced to $1 million when new budgetary demands were placed by other NCI divisions. Approximately 30 serious inquiries about the RFP were made to NCI officials, and 12 completed proposals were received in the NCI office by the deadline, which was formally extended past the six weeks originally granted because of the strong protests of several hospice planners that the time allowed for the preparation of proposals was far too short.

The 1976 RFP included a 75-page description of the criteria for the requested proposals, along with seven major attachments and many pages of instructions to whomever was offering. The entire RFP was couched in the legal terms of a huge contract.

The 1976 RFP specifically disallowed proposals from hospitals because, according to Mr. Burke, NCI officials did not want to fund hospitals whose principle intent was to find money for unused beds. The latest RFP also made it clear that care for terminal patients (not candidates for rehabilitation services) was being requested. Thus NCI, as a matter of low priority, without excessive speed, and with a maximum of red tape that tended to impede, rather than encourage, the development of hospices, made its first significant effort to pay for some care of a relatively small number of terminal cancer victims in a very few American cities. Site visits by NCI bureaucrats have been made to a number of the prospective developers (including a winter trip to the one in Hawaii), and it appears likely that the total of three or four hospices that were originally intended for funding have been reduced to one or two.

One of the most interesting aspects of the NCI response to the hospice movement concerns the reasons why the response has been so slow. Are hospices threatening to NCI officials? What is it, specifically, that arouses opposition? Or, in a less extreme sense, why are hospices not considered sufficiently significant to engender a widespread and enthusiastic federal response?

As described in this book the effect of death on culture and the reluctance of many members of our society to confront directly the probability of death makes it difficult to bring the hospice concept to reality. There is also the notion that hospitals meet the legitimate needs of dying people so that we do not have to deal directly with death. There is a strong orientation within NCI towards research and preventive measures, and a large number of other factors mitigate against a strong and supportive public role in the development of hospices across the country. Hospices, of course, are an innovation within the health care delivery industry. They are not the usual technological innovation that researchers are used to studying. Hospices are, instead, an important organizational innovation.

I suggest that the institutional lag demonstrated by the NCI response to the hospice movement be subjected to research. Interesting hypotheses that could be examined by social scientists who are interested in the failure to adopt an organizational innovation, as suggested in this book, include the following:

1. Organizational innovation is negatively correlated to age; the older the NCI official, the less likely he or she is to be receptive to the introduction of an innovation such as hospices.

2. The recruitment of NCI policymakers from among older physicians, as well as the substantial tenure and long-term career patterns associated with the NCI bureaucracy are likely to result in resistance to organizational innovation.

3. The generalized concern of a bureaucracy (and especially one composed of people who consider themselves general oncologists or staff concerned with a wide-scale war on cancer) is likely to result in a greater resistance to organizational innovation than

would be evidenced by people who considered themselves narrow, interdependent specialists.

4. The discrepancy in backgrounds between NCI decision makers, on the one hand, and leaders of the hospice movement (who are often ministers, nursing home administrators, activist citizens, victims of cancer, and planners of various sorts), on the other, is likely to make it difficult for proponents of hospices to convince the well-established professionals of the worth and validity of their cause.

5. Hospices represent a somewhat radical critique of existing medical and hospital practices, and the implied criticism of the status quo is likely to engender opposition.

6. The consideration of hospices forces a bureaucratic analyst to also consider directly a subject (death) that has remained largely taboo in our culture, and this subtle aspect of hospice proposals makes such proposals somewhat distasteful.

Thus physicians, bureaucrats, planners and legislators do not have to examine merely an organizational innovation when considering a hospice proposal, but also our society's views on death. We are not discussing *any* institution newly proposed for funding. We are talking about death, how we manage it and fail to manage it properly.

A more comprehensive model of institutional lag as it affects the development of hospices would have to include at least the following new elements:

In the public sector:

Failure of the federal Executive Branch to perceive the importance of the issue or the relevant service gap, or to establish a policy planning mechanism that deals with death and dying

Failure of the Legislative branch to perceive large-scale public support for the new innovation or to provide any mandate to Congressional committees to consider the impact of federal policies on the quality of death in America

Failure of bureaucratic initiative to allocate a high priority to the innovation in a competitive situation of relatively scarce resources

In the private sector:

Institutional investments already in place, particularly in hospitals, which are threatened by an organizational innovation

Failure of medical education to confront the issues concerned with the termination of human life

Tendency of many physicians already in private practice to pursue life-preserving techniques and then to abandon the patient when those techniques fail, as if responsibility for service ends when the hope for longevity ends

Proclivity of industry and other sources in the private sector to support established practices rather than innovation by their multibillion dollar donations

On a community basis:

Failure of the many agencies and voluntary organizations supporting the extensive public health service network to provide services to dying and bereaving people

Failure of organizations not primarily concerned with medical issues but concerned with issues of social responsibility to perceive the neglect of those who are dying

Failure of local governments to appreciate the large-scale service gap that leaves local agencies unable to respond to the needs of the dying

On an individual basis:

Socioculturally induced tendency to deny the inevitability
of our own deaths
Tendency, perhaps as a part of that personal denial, to
largely ignore the deaths of others

The development of a network of hospices across the
nation encounters not so much an opposition as a reluctance on a grand scale that prefers to take a form that
social scientists call institutional lag. There are cultural,
psychological, institutional, and financial reasons why we
feel more comfortable not confronting the issues that hospices force upon us. That forcing continues inexorably
(partly because people continue to die miserable deaths,
and some people persist in caring about that misery), but
there are many institutions in our society that perceive an
interest in slowing it down. Until the interests of the dying
and their families are recognized as universal concerns
that affect the last stage of all our lives and the quality of
life in our society, we as a nation will continue to die
miserable deaths.

Notes

Chapter 1

1. Definition submitted to staffs of other hospice development groups in a private memo dated 2/4/76 from Dennis Rezendes of Hospice, Inc., New Haven, Connecticut and which was later submitted to several Congressional staff members.

2. Whitehead, Anthony. *In the service of old age: The welfare of psychogeriatric patients.* Pelican, p. 59.

3. Dobihal, Edward. Talk or terminal care? *Connecticut Medicine,* 1974, *38,* 365.

4. Kohn, Judith. Hospice movement provides humane alternative for terminally ill patients. *Modern Healthcare,* 1976, 26.

5. Quoted by Knon, Joan. Designing a better place to die. *New York,* March 1, 1976, 43.

6. Holden, Constance. Hospices: For the dying, relief from pain and fear. *Science,* 1976, *193,* 389.

7. Private minutes of Hospice Symposium Planning Sessions, comprised of 14 hospice developers from institutions and held on July 28, 1976.

8. Quotations from *Referral: Hospice* written and published by Hospice, Inc., New Haven, Connecticut.

9. Craven, Joan, & Wald, Florence. Hospice care for dying patients. *American Journal of Nursing,* 1975, *75,* 1821.

Chapter 2

1. This section adheres closely to the data and analysis presented in Speigelman, Mortimer. *Significant mortality and morbidity trends in the United States since 1900.* Bryn Mawr: American College of Life Underwriters, 1966.

2. *Ibid.*

3. *Ibid.,* p. 2, taken from the Bureau of the Census and the National Center for Health Statistics.

4. *Ibid.*

5. *Ibid.,* from various reports of the National Center for Health Statistics.

6. Speigelman, Mortimer. *Ensuring medical care for the aged.* Pension Research Council, Wharton School of Finance and Commerce by Richard Irwin, Inc., 1960, p. 5. This section on the aged follows this book closely.

7. *Ibid.,* p. 6.

8. American Cancer Society. *1976 cancer facts and figures,* p. 13.

9. U.S. Department of Health, Education and Welfare Vital Health Statistics. *Mortality trends for leading causes of death, United States,* 1950–1969, Series 20, Number 16, see especially pp. 1–7.

10. American Cancer Society, *1976 cancer facts and figures,* p. 12.

11. This discussion of racial differences follows closely Seidman, Herbert, Silverberg, Edwin, & Holleb, Arthur. *Cancer statistics, 1976, A comparison of white and black populations.* American Cancer Society, 1976, p. 4.

12. *Ibid.,* p. 12.

13. *Ibid.,* p. 13.

14. This section on the NCI report is taken from Schmeck, Harold. Environmental factors in cancer are hinted in atlas on

nonwhites in the *New York Times,* January 6, 1977, p. 18 and the AP Report printed in the *Miami Herald,* same date, p. 11-AW.

15. This section on the unreliability of certain cancer statistics is taken from a special *Newsday* report reprinted in *The Ithaca Journal,* January 22, 1977, p. 2.

Chapter 3

1. The author is aware of the inadequacies in the English language which make it awkward to use the masculine and feminine pronouns together. They should be understood as interchangeable throughout, and they will be alternated in this book.

2. Kastenbaum & Aisenberg, *The psychology of death,* New York: Springer Publishing Company, 1972, p. 7.

3. Issner, Natalie. Can the child be distracted from his disease? Presented to the National Conference on Human Values and Cancer, June 22–24, 1972, in Atlanta, Georgia.

4. Schowalter, John. The child's reaction to his own terminal illness. In Schoenberg, et al. *Loss and grief: Psychological management on medical practice.* New York: Columbia University Press, 1970, pp. 51–69.

5. *Ibid.,* p. 52.

6. Wiener, Jerry. Reaction of the family to the fatal illness of a child. In Schoenberg, et al. *Loss and grief,* p. 87.

7. *Ibid.,* p. 89.

8. Kastenbaum & Aisenberg, *The psychology of death,* p. 41.

9. For an excellent review, see *Ibid.,* pp. 65–112, which form the basis for this paragraph.

10. Schoenberg, Bernard, & Senescu, Robert. The patient's reactions to fatal illness. In Schoenberg, et al., *Loss and grief,* p. 222.

11. Titchner, J. L. et al. Problems of delay in seeking surgical care. *Journal of the American Medical Association,* 1956, *160,* 1187.

12. Aitken-Swan, J., & Paterson, R. The cancer patient: delay in treatment. *British Medical Journal,* 1955, *00,* 623.

13. Fisher, S. Motivation for patient delay. *Archives of General Psychiatry,* 1967, *16,* 676.

14. Hammerschlag, C. A., et al. Breast symptoms and patient delay: psychological variables involved. *Cancer,* 1964, *17,* 1480.

15. Hinton, John. The influence of previous personality on reactions to having terminal cancer. Paper prepared for a conference on Death Research: Methods and Substance, Berkeley, California, March 21–23, 1973, and published in *Omega, The Journal of Death and Dying,* 1975, *6,* 95–111.

16. Schoenberg & Senescu. The patient's reactions, pp. 224, 225.

17. *Ibid.,* pp. 226, 227.

18. *Ibid.,* p. 227.

19. *Ibid.,* p. 228.

20. *Ibid.,* pp. 229–230.

21. Rosenblatt, Paul, Jackson, Douglas, & Walsh, Rose. Coping with anger and aggression in mourning. *Omega, The Journal of Death and Dying,* 1975, *6,* 271–282.

22. *Ibid.,* p. 271.

23. *Ibid.*

24. *Ibid.,* p. 281.

25. Erickson, Ralph. Hacking it. *P.T.A. Magazine,* 1974, *69,* 26–27.

26. *U. S. News and World Report,* April 5, 1974, pp. 59–60. The statistics in this paragraph are from this article.

27. Kutscher, Austin. Practical aspects of bereavement. In Schoenberg, et al., *Loss and grief,* p. 281.

28. *Ibid.,* pp. 283–285.

29. Shneidman, E. S. Orientations towards death. In White, R. W. (Ed.). *The study of lives.* New York: Atherton Press, 1963, p. 201.

30. Schoenberg, & Senescu. The patient's reactions, p. 233.

31. Gonda, Thomas. Pain and addiction in terminal illness. In Schoenberg, et al. *Loss and grief,* p. 262.

32. Twycross, Robert. Clinical experience with diamorphine in advanced malignant disease. *International Journal of Clinical Pharmacology,* 1974, *00,* 198.

33. *Ibid.*

34. *Ibid.*

35. Glaser, Barbey, & Strauss, Anselm. *Awareness of dying.* Aldive, 1965.

36. Glaser, Barbey, & Strauss, Anselm. Awareness of dying. In Schoenberg, et al. *Loss and grief,* p. 305.

37. Kubler-Ross, Elizabeth. *On death and dying.* New York: Macmillan, 1969.

38. Schulz, Richard, & Aderman, David. Clinical research and the stages of dying. *Omega, The Journal of Death and Dying,* 1974, *5.*

39. *Ibid.*

40. Wiener, Jerry. Response of medical personnel to the fatal illness of a child. In Schoenberg, et al. *Loss and grief,* p. 103.

41. Schoenberg & Senescu. The patient's reactions, p. 221.

42. *Ibid.,* pp. 231–232.

43. Schoenberg, Bernard. Management of a dying patient. In Schoenberg, et al., *Loss and grief,* pp. 238–260.

44. Strauss & Glaser. Awareness of dying. In Schoenberg, et al. *Loss and grief,* p. 299.

45. *Ibid.,* pp. 307–308.

46. Kastenbaum, Robert. Towards standards of care for the terminally ill, part II: What standards exist today? *Omega, The Journal of Death and Dying,* 1975, *6,* 289, 290.

47. Heimlich, Henry, & Kutscher, Austin. The family's reaction to terminal illness. In Schoenberg et al., *Loss and grief,* pp. 275–279.

48. Dubrey, Sister Rita Jean, & Terril, Laura. The loneliness of the dying person: An exploratory study. *Omega, The Journal of Death and Dying,* 1975, *6,* 357–371.

49. Kastenbaum & Aisenberg, *The psychology of death,* p. 217.

50. *Ibid.,* p. 215.

51. *Ibid.,* 221–222.

52. Quint, Jeanne. The social contest of dying. Presentation at the Conference on Terminal Illness and Impending Death Among the Aged, Washington, D. C., May 10, 1966, quoted in *Ibid.,* p. 224.

53. *Ibid.,* pp. 209–214.

54. *Ibid.,* pp. 225–230.

55. *Ibid.,* p. 230.

56. Duff, Raymond, & Hollingshead, August. *Sickness and society.* New York: Harper and Row, 1968.

57. Kastenberg & Aisenbaum, *The psychology of death,* p. 191. This section of this chapter is based heavily on their book, pp. 191–250.

58. *Ibid.,* pp. 192–193.

59. *Ibid.,* p. 205.

60. *Ibid.,* pp. 240, 241.

61. *Ibid.,* pp. 241, 242.

Chapter 4

1. Information in this section of this chapter is taken from Wald, Florence, Caring in terminal illness, an address delivered to the *Inauguration of the School of Nursing and Installation of Dean Loretta Ford,* December 8 and 9, 1972, University of Rochester, Rochester, New York, and included in the *Proceedings* of that Inauguration and Installation, published privately by the University of Rochester.

2. *Ibid.,* p. 51.

3. *Ibid.,* p. 52.

4. *Ibid.*

5. *Ibid.*

6. *Ibid.,* p. 54.

7. *Ibid.*

8. *Ibid.,* p. 55.

9. *Ibid.,* p. 56.

10. Some of the design plans for Hospice Inc., as well as an interview with Mr. Chan, are included in Kron, Joan, Designing a better place to die. *New York,* 1976, 43–49.

11. *Ibid.,* p. 49.

12. Wald, Florence, *Caring in terminal illness,* p. 57.

13. *Ibid.,* p. 59.

14. Saunders, Cicely. Components of Hospice Care. *Hospice Care and Cancer,* in press.

Chapter 5

1. This chapter relies heavily on a number of very valuable unpublished reports and on-site visits to St. Christopher's Hospice by Americans during the past three years. Most especially, I am indebted to Claire Ravizza, Hospice Coordinator of Rochester Cancer Center, Strong Memorial Hospital, Rochester, New York for her unpublished site-visit report prepared after she spent three weeks at St. Christopher's in 1976. Her reports, and the opportunities she gave me to interview her at great length, form the primary basis for the chapter. In addition, I used a lengthy letter from Dr. Cicely Saunders, founder of St. Christopher's, which criticized Ms. Ravizza's site visit report. I am also indebted to Dr. Leonard Liegner, Professor of Radiology at the College of Physicians and Surgeons, New York City, and the Chief of Radiation Therapy at St. Luke's Hospital Center, and Presbyterian Hospital, both in New York City, who wrote a lengthy report after a 1974 site visit to St. Christopher's. His report was particularly helpful in preparing the section on pain relief. The final major debt I want to acknowledge in the preparation of this chapter is to Dr. Cicely Saunders herself, who wrote a chapter tentatively entitled "The Working of St. Christopher's" for a Foundation of Thanatology book, as yet unpublished, tentatively titled *Medical Care of the Dying Patient.* Dr. Saunders' writings, both in the chapter and in various St. Christophers' publications which I had at my disposal, as well as her comments on various American site visits, have provided extremely useful insights. St. Christopher's also publishes Annual Re-

ports, which I have used here, and which include detailed reports from the directors of each department and admissions and referral statistics along with account summaries for expenditures and income. While a number of magazine and newspaper articles on St. Christopher's have appeared in the popular press in recent years, along with several house-published pamphlets and brochures, virtually all of which I have examined, all the data available to the interested researcher is contained in the major sources I have listed above. These sources, both the published and private reports, and especially Ms. Ravizza's unpublished site visit report, serve as the foundation for the present chapter, and the statistics presented in the concluding tables are taken from a summary of St. Christopher's annual reports.

Chapter 6

1. Hospice—what it is: Board of Directors, Hospice, Inc., New Haven, Connecticut.

2. Dobihal, Edward F., Jr. Talk or terminal care? *Connecticut Medicine, 38,* 1974, 367.

3. McCormack, Patricia. Helping hands, hearts for terminally ill. *The Hartford Times,* March 14, 1976.

4. The first 18 members of the Board of Directors are:

   Mrs. George M. Allen, Community Leader, Hamden, CT.

   Mrs. Marilyn Beach, Associate Director of Inpatient Nursing, Yale-New Haven Hospital, New Haven, CT.

   Mr. Roland Bixler, President, J.B.T. Instruments, New Haven, CT.

   Father Robert Canny, Clinical Pastoral Education Supervisor, St. Raphael's Hospital, Director of Hospitals —Archdiosis of Hartford, New Haven, CT.

   George Cohn, M.D., Chief, Consultation, Psychosomatic and Liaison Services, Veterans Administration Hospital, New Haven, CT.

   Dean Donna K. Diers, Yale School of Nursing, New Haven, CT.

Rev. Edward F. Dobihal, Jr., Director, Department of Religious Ministries, Yale-New Haven Hospital, New Haven, CT.

Mr. James Gilbert, President, C. W. Blakeslee and Sons, Inc., New Haven, CT.

Ira Goldenberg, M.D., Professor of Clinical Surgery, Yale-New Haven Hospital, New Haven, CT.

Mrs. William Horowitz, New Haven, CT.

Mrs. Henry H. Pierce, New Haven, CT.

Mr. Walter Ramshaw, Acting Chief, Cooperative Studies Center, Veterans Administration Hospital, New Haven, CT.

Mr. Cornell Scott, M.P.H., Project Director, Hill Health Center, New Haven, CT.

Mr. Stanley Trotman, District Manager, Northwestern Mutual Insurance, New Haven, CT.

Mr. Henry P. Wald, P.E., Director of Health Science Planning, Columbia University, College of Physicians and Surgeons, New Haven, CT.

Morris Wessel, M.D., Pediatrician, New Haven, CT.

Mrs. Howell White, New Haven, CT.

Mr. Frank Wollensack, General Manager, Operation-Plans, SNET Co., New Haven, CT.

5. Kron, Joan. Designing a better place to die. *New York,* 1976, 47.

6. Endorsements of Hospice by Connecticut and New Haven agencies included the following. (All agencies are located in New Haven, Connecticut.)

American Cancer Society, New Haven Metro Unit: Saul Goldberg, Chairman, Service and Rehabilitation Center

Association of Community Health Service Agencies, Inc.: Board of Directors

The Auxiliary Yale-New Haven Hospital: Board of Managers

Community Health Care Plan: I. S. Falk, Executive
Director

Connecticut Conference of the United Church of Christ:
Samual W. Fogal, Chairman

Connecticut Hospital Planning Commission, Inc.:
William T. McClintock, Associate Director

Connecticut League for Nursing: Mary B. Heath,
President

The Connecticut Mental Health Center: Boris M.
Astrachan, M.D., Director

Connecticut Nurses Association, Inc.: Carol D. DeYoung,
Executive Director

Connecticut Regional Medical Program: Edward F.
Morrissey, Acting Director

The Connecticut Society of Internal Medicine Council

Danbury Hospital Auxiliary: Mrs. Kathleen Hannakin,
President

Davenport Residence Inc.: Board of Directors

Most Rev. Joseph F. Donelly, D.D.

The Downtown Cooperative Ministry, Inc.: The Board

The Episcopal Church: John M. Allin, Presiding Bishop

First United Methodist Church of West Haven: William
J. Baugh, Pastor

The Gaylord Hospital: Alice Moore, Director of Social
Service

Griffin Hospital: A. J. Deluca, Administrator; James H.
Moore, Director, Department of Community Health

The Hospital of St. Raphael: Sister Louise Anthony,
Administrator; Carolyn Glenn, Continuing Care Director

Jewish Family Service of New Haven, Inc.: Irwin I.
Goldberg, Executive Director

Junior League of New Haven, Inc.: Mrs. Philip B. Cowles,
Jr., President

Mental Health Association of Connecticut, Inc.: Board of
Directors

New Britain Area Conference of Churches: Board of
Directors

Orange Public Health Nursing Service: Patricia Zeoli,
Chairman of the Board

Quinnipiac College, Faculty of the School of Allied
Health and Natural Sciences: Stanley S. Katz, Dean

Regional Visiting Nurse Agency, Inc.: Margory
Richardson, Executive Director for the Board

Rehabilitation Center: Albert P. Calli, Executive Director

Rehabilitation Council of Greater New Haven: Dr.
Robert G. LaCamera, Chairman

Sage Advocates Programs: Brenda J. Stiers, Director

South Central Connecticut Comprehensive Health
Planning, Inc.: Board of Directors

Veterans Administration Hospital, West Haven: Willis O.
Underwood, Hospital Director; Sarah S. Isenberg, Public
Health Clinician

Visiting Nurse Association of New Haven: Jane D.
Keeler, Executive Director

Yale-New Haven Hospital: Board of Directors (Minutes,
April 25, 1973)

Yale-New Haven Hospital: Mrs. Angus Gordon,
Chairman; Committee on the Role of the Hospital in
Addressing Community Health Needs

Yale-New Haven Hospital: Mary C. Sayers, Home Care
Coordinator; Robert W. Harrison, Chief, Medical Social
Work

Yale University Divinity School: Deal Colin Williams

Yale University Health Services: Joseph Axelrod,
Administrator

Yale University School of Medicine: Joseph R. Bertino,
Professor of Medicine and Pharmacology; Fredrick C.
Redlich, Professor of Psychiatry; Ronald R. Rozett,
Assistant Professor of Medicine

Yale University School of Nursing: Donna Diers, Dean

7. From personal notes of Claire Ravizza from interview with Florence Wald, July 21, 1975.

8. Referral: Hospice. Published by Hospice, Inc., New Haven, Connecticut.

9. Dobihal, Edward. Press release, October, 1974.

10. Friends of Hospice, news from hospice. p. 3.

11. Wald, Florence. Caring in terminal illness. An address delivered to the *Inauguration of the School of Nursing and Installation of Dean Loretta Ford,* December 8 and 9, 1972, University of Rochester, Rochester, New York, and included in the *Proceedings* of that Inauguration and Installation, published privately by the University of Rochester.

12. Friends of Hospice, news from hospice.

13. Notes from home care workshop conducted by Dr. Sylvia Lack at the First National Hospice Symposium in Branford, Connecticut, October 27, 1975.

14. *Ibid.*

15. *Ibid.*

16. At home with death. *Newsweek,* 1/6/75, p. 43.

17. Death with dignity—at home. *The Washington Post,* November 16, 1975.

18. Kron, Joan. Designing a better place to die, p. 47. The physical description of Hospice, Inc. is taken mainly from the plans contained in this article.

19. *Ibid.,* p. 48.

20. Hospice. Newsletter published by Hospice, Inc., New Haven, Connecticut, Volume III, No. 1, p. 1.

21. *Ibid.,* p. 3.

22. The preceeding data and information came from the submission filed with the Connecticut Commission on Hospitals by Hospice, Inc. and from *Ibid.*

23. Hospice, Inc., Hospice.

24. *Ibid.*

25. Notes by Claire Ravizza from an interview with Florence Wald, July 21, 1975.

Chapter 7

1. From personal tapes of the author's interviews with Claire Ravizza, November 3 and 4, 1978.

2. Patterson, W. B. Memorandum to Division of Oncology Clinicians, May 21, 1973, p. 1.

3. *Ibid.*

4. Patterson, W. B. Letter to A. Sharleen Bruse, Executive Director, Monroe County Cancer and Leukemia Association, November 19, 1974, pp. 1, 2.

5. Patterson, W. B. Letter to Barbara Zartman, President of Euthanasia Educational Council, May 29, 1974, p. 1.

6. Davenport-Hatch Foundation letter to W. B. Patterson, November 19, 1974, p. 1.

7. *Ibid.*

8. From the author's taped interview with Claire Ravizza, November 3 and 4, 1978.

9. *Ibid.*

10. Ravizza, Claire, interim report to M.C.C.L.A., January 9, 1976.

11. *Ibid.*

12. From the author's taped interview with Claire Ravizza, November 3 and 4, 1978.

13. *Ibid.*

14. Ravizza, Claire, interim report to M.C.C.L.A., January 9, 1976.

15. Ravizza, Claire, notes from interview with Marilyn Weiser, October 22, 1975.

16. Ravizza, Claire, interim report to M.C.C.L.A., January 9, 1976.

17. From the author's taped interview with Claire Ravizza, November 3 and 4, 1978.

18. Demonstration and training in hospice care. From Cancer Control Contract submitted to National Cancer Institute by University of Rochester Cancer Center, pp. 214–216.

19. From the author's taped interview with Claire Ravizza, No-
    vember 3 and 4, 1978.
20. *Ibid.*

Chapter 8

1. Cities that now have hospice planning groups include the
   following:

California

> Berkeley, Caguiva Hills, Canoga Park, Kentfield, Los Ange-
> les, Oakland, Palo Alto, Pasadena, Redwood City, San
> Diego, San Francisco, San Jose, Santa Barbara, Seal Beach,
> Solara Beach, Tiburon, Walnut Creek

Colorado

> Colorado Springs, Denver

Connecticut

> Farmington, Hamden, Manchester, New Haven, Newing-
> ton, Wallingford

Florida

> Clearwater, Orlando

Hawaii

> Honolulu

Illinois

> Chicago, Evanston, Glencoe, Park Ridge, Wheaton

Indiana

> Notre Dame

Maine

> Blue Hills Farms, Westbrook

Maryland

> Baltimore, Catonsville

Massachusetts

> Boston, Brookline, Fall River, New Bedford, Newton, Wayland

Michigan

> Detroit

Minnesota

> Minneapolis, Rochester

Missouri

> Kansas City, St. Louis

Nevada

> Las Vegas

New Hampshire

> Manchester, Salem

New Jersey

> Boonton, Dover, Dunellen, Flemington, Morristown, Newark, Princeton, Rockaway, Summit, Trenton

New Mexico

> Las Vegas

New York

> Binghamton, Buffalo, Corning, East Meadow, Hastings-on-Hudson, New Hyde Park, New York City, Rochester, Rye, Spring Valley, White Plains

North Carolina

> Durham

North Dakota

> Fargo

Ohio

> Cogun Falls, Cincinnati, Cleveland

Pennsylvania

Danville, Harrisburg, King of Prussia, Philadelphia

Rhode Island

Providence

Vermont

Burlington

Virginia

Falls Creek, Richmond

Washington

Seattle, Tacoma

Washington, D.C.

Wisconsin

Milwaukee

Canada

Montreal

Chapter 9

1. This introductory section is based directly on the 1975 revised edition of *The National Cancer Institute,* published by the U. S. Department of Health, Education and Welfare (No. NIH 76-792), and on other introductory literature available to the public from NCI.

2. This description of the Council is taken and adapted from *Research and Related Programs of the National Cancer Institute,* Public Health Service Publication No. 458-A, revised in 1969, p. 10.

3. Developed from charts in the National Cancer Institute Fact Book, p. 25.

4. Taken directly from NIH 76-792, pp. 25–26.

5. *Ibid.,* p. 27.

6. *Ibid.,* p. 28.

7. *Ibid.,* p. 47.
8. *Ibid.,* p. 30.
9. Derived from *Ibid.,* p. 47.
10. Taken and adapted from Public Health Service No. 458-A, pp. 12–13.
11. This description of the Cancer Control Program is adapted from the *Appendices to the National Cancer Program Operational Plan,* August, 1974, DHEW No. NIH 75-778, pp. B.1-1 to B.3-4.
12. Lawrence Burke, in two conversations with the author in interviews conducted in late November, 1976 and December 22, 1976.
13. Title of the 1974 RFP, furnished by HEW/NIH/NCI.
14. Burke, in conversation with the author.
15. 1974 RFP, p. 4.
16. *Ibid.,* p. 7.
17. *Ibid.,* p. 4.
18. *Ibid.,* p. 5.
19. *Ibid.*
20. "Exhibit A, Scope of Work," attached to RFP, Ibid., pp. 27–28.
21. Implementation of the 'hospice' concept for the care of terminal cancer patients. HEW/NIH/NCI RFP No. N01-CN-65375-05, dated March 29, 1976.

Bibliography

Abrahamsson, H. *The origin of death: Studies in African mythology.* Uppsala: Studia Ethnographica Upsaliensia, 1951.

Abrams, R. D., & Finesinger, J. R. Guilt reactions in patients with cancer. *Cancer,* 1953, *6,* 474–482.

Abrams, R. D., Jameson, G., Poehlman, M., & Snyder, S. Terminal care in cancer. *New England Medical Journal,* 1945, *232,* 719–724.

Acri, M. J. & Miller, A. J. *Death: A bibliographical guide.* Metuchen, N.J.: Scarecrow Press, 1977. A thorough bibliography that lists thanatologic works under the headings of education, humanities, medical profession and nursing, religion and theology, science, social sciences, and audiovisual media.

Addiss, L. K. The family in today's economic world. In *Catastrophic illness: Impact on families, challenge to the professions,* symposium proceedings. New York: Cancer Care, Inc. of the National Cancer Foundation, 1966.

Advocate for Human Services: A bi-weekly Washington roundup of legislation and activities affecting social work and people. Washington, D.C.: National Association of Social Workers.

Agee, J. *A death in the family.* New York: Avon, 1963.

Aitken-Swan, J. Nursing the late cancer patient at home. *Practitioner,* 1959, *183,* 64–69.

Aitken-Swan, J., & Easson, E. C. Reactions of cancer patients on being told their diagnosis. *British Medical Journal,* 1959, *1,* 779–783.

Alderson, M. R. Terminal care in malignant disease. *British Journal of Preventive and Social Medicine,* 1970, *24,* 120–123.

Aldrich, C. K. Dying patient's grief. *Journal of the American Medical Association,* 1963, *329.*

Aldrich, C. K. Emotional problems in catastrophic illness. In *Catastrophic illness: Impact on families, challenge to the professions,* symposium proceedings, New York: Cancer Care Inc. of the National Cancer Foundation, 1966.

Aldwinckle, R. F. *Death in the secular city.* London: G. Allen, 1972.

Alsop, S. *Stay of execution.* Philadelphia: Lippincott, 1973.

American Medical Association. *Statement on home health care.* Chicago, American Medical Association, 1973.

Andersen, R. People and their hospital insurance: Comparisons of the uninsured, those with one policy, and those with multiple coverage. Chicago: Center for Health Administration, University of Chicago, Research Series 23, 1967.

Anderson, C. Aspects of pathological grief and mourning. *International Journal of Psychoanalysis,* 1949, *30,* 48–55.

Anthony, S. *Discovery of death in childhood and after.* New York: Basic Books, 1972.

Aries, P. *Western attitudes toward death.* Baltimore: Johns Hopkins University Press, 1974.

Aronson, G. J. Treatment of the dying patient. In H. Feifel (Ed.), *The meaning of death.* New York: McGraw-Hill, 1959, chap. 14.

Ashton, P. Health security program: Medicine in the free enterprise system. *Vital Speeches,* 1970, *37,* 100–102.

Bailey, M. A survey of the social needs of patients with incurable lung cancer. *Almoner,* 1959, *11,* 379–391.

Barckley, V. Enough time for good nursing. *Nursing Outlook,* 1964, *12,* 44–48.

Bard, M. The sequence of emotional reactions in radical mastectomy patients. *Public Health Reports,* 1952, *67,* 1144–1148.

Bard, M., & Sutherland, A. M. Psychological impact of cancer and its treatment: IV—adaptation to radical mastectomy. *Cancer,* 1956, *9,* 1120.

Barry, H., Jr. Significance of maternal bereavement before age of eight in psychiatric patients. *Archives of Neurological Psychiatry,* 1949, *62,* 630–637.

Bartlett, H. Frontiers of medical social work. *Social Work,* 1962, *7,* 2.

Becker, A. H., & Weisman, A. D. The patient with a fatal illness —to tell or not to tell. *Journal of the American Medical Association,* 1967, *201,* 646–648.

Becker, E. *The denial of death.* New York: Collier-Macmillan, 1973.

Becker, H. S., et al. *Boys in white: Student culture in medical school.* Chicago: University of Chicago Press, 1961.

Beigler, J. S. Anxiety as an aid in the prognostication of impending death. *Archives of Neurology and Psychiatry,* 1957, *77,* 171–177.

Bellak, L. (Ed.). *Psychology of physical illness.* New York: Grune & Stratton, 1952.

Benda, C. E. Bereavement and grief work. *Journal of Pastoral Care,* 1962, *16,* 1–13.

Benjamin, B. Bereavement and heart disease. *Journal of Biosocial Science,* 1971, *3,* 61–67.

Bergler, E. Psychopathology and duration of mourning in neurotics. *Journal of Clinical Psychopathology,* 1948, *3,* 48–82.

Bergman, A. B., & Schulte, C. J. (Eds.). Care of the child with cancer. *Pediatrics* (Suppl), 1967, *40,* 487.

Berki, S. E. National health insurance: An idea whose time has come. *Annals of the American Academy of Political and Social Science CCCXCIX,* 1972, *1,* 125–144.

Berle, B., Pinsky, R. H., Wolf, S., & Wolf, H. G. A clinical guide to prognosis in stress diseases. *Journal of the American Medical Association,* 1952, *149,* 1624–1628.

Bermann, E. *Scapegoat: The impact of a death on an American family.* Ann Arbor, Michigan: University of Michigan Press, 1973.

Blenkner, M., Beggs, H. *Home aide service and the aged: A controlled study, part II: The service program.* Cleveland, Ohio: Benjamin Rose Institute, 1970.

Blewett, L. J. To die at home. *Journal of Nursing,* 1970, 2602–2604.

Bowers, M. K., Jackson, E., Knight, J., & LeShan, L. *Counseling the dying.* New York: Nelson, 1964.

Bowlby, J. Grief and mourning in infancy and early childhood. *Psychoanalytic Study of the Child,* 1960, *15,* 9–52.

Bowlby, J. Childhood mourning and its implications for psychiatry. *American Journal of Psychiatry,* 1960, *118,* 481–498.

Bowlby, J. Processes of mourning. *International Journal of Psychoanalysis,* 1961, *42,* 317–40.

Boyle, K. *Death of a man.* Rahway, N.J.: Quinn and Boden, 1936.

Bohrod, M. G. Uses of the autopsy. *Journal of the American Medical Association,* 1965, *193,* 810–812.

Bozeman, M. F., Orbach, C. E., & Sutherland, A. M. Psychological impact of cancer and its treatment. Part III. *Cancer,* 1955, *8,* 1–19.

Brauer, P. H. Should the patient be told the truth? *Nursing Outlook,* 1960, *8,* 672–676.

Brim, O. G. Jr., Freeman, H. E., Levine, S., & Scotch, N. A. *The dying patient.* New York: Russell Sage Foundation, 1970.

Brown, F. Depression and childhood bereavement. *Journal of Mental Science,* 1961, *107,* 754–77.

Burns, T., & Stalker, G. M. *The management of innovation.* London: Tavistock, 1961.

Busse, E. W. The problems of aging and the homebound: An overview. Durham, N.C.: The Church's Ministry to the Homebound, Report on a Seminar on Visiting the Homebound, 1965.

Busse, E. W. Psychophysiological reactions and psychoneurotic disorders related to physical changes in the elderly. *Proceedings of the Eighth International Congress of Gerontology,* 1969, *1,* 195–197.

Cain, A. C., et al. Children's disturbed reactions to the death of a sibling. *American Journal of Orthopsychiatry,* 1959, *34,* 2.

Caine, L. *Widow.* New York: Morrow, 1974.

Cancer Care, Inc. of the National Cancer Foundation. *Report of a symposium on terminal illness.* New York: National Cancer Foundation, 1956.

Cancer Care, Inc. of the National Cancer Foundation. *A constructive approach to terminal illness,* symposium proceedings. New York: National Cancer Foundation, 1958.

Cancer Care, Inc. of the National Cancer Foundation. *Catastrophic illness: impact on families, challenge to the professions,* symposium proceedings. New York: National Cancer Foundation, 1966.

Cancer Care, Inc. of the National Cancer Foundation. *Catastrophic illness in the seventies: Critical issues and complex decisions,* proceedings of the fourth national symposium. New York: National Cancer Foundation, 1966.

Cancer statistics, 1976, A comparison of white and black populations. New York: American Cancer Society, 1976.

Caplan, G. *Support systems and community mental health.* New York: Behavioral Publications, 1974.

Cappon, D. The psychology of dying. *Pastoral Psychology,* 1960, *12,* 35–44.

Capron, A. M., & Kass, L. R. A statutory definition of the standards for determining human death: An appraisal and a proposal. *University of Pennsylvania Law Review,* 1972, *121,* 87–118.

Carr, A. A lifetime of preparation for bereavement. *Archives of Thanatology,* 1969, *1,* 14–18.

Cartwright, A., et al. *Life before death.* Boston: Routledge and Kegan, 1973.

Cassell, E. J. Learning to Die. *Bulletin of the New York Academy of Medicine,* 1973, *49,* 12.

Choron, J. *Death and modern man.* New York: Collier Books, 1971.

Clayton, P., Halikes, J. A., & Maurice, W. L. The bereavement of the widowed. *Diseases of the Nervous System,* 1971.

Cobb, B. Psychological impact of long illness and death of a child on the family circle. *Journal of Pediatrics,* 1956, *49,* 746–51.

Cockerill, E. A social view of terminal illness. A constructive approach to terminal illness, symposium proceedings. New York: Cancer Care, Inc. of the National Cancer Foundation, 1958.

Committee for Economic Development, Building a National Health Care System, A statement by the Research and Policy Committee, New York, 1973.

Committee Print (Special Committee on Aging, United States Senate). Alternatives to nursing home care: A proposal with discussion of deficiencies in federally-assisted programs for treatment of long-term disability. Washington, D.C.: U.S. Gov't Ptg. Off., 1971.

Cooper, E. F. A constructive approach to irreversible illness. *The Journal of Jewish Communal Service,* 1959, *36,* 2.

Cotter, Z. M., Sr. Institutional care of the terminally ill. *Hospital Progress,* 1971.

Cox, P. R., & Ford, J. R. The mortality of widows shortly after widowhood. *Lancet,* 1964, *1,* 163–164.

Cramond, W. A. Psychotherapy of the dying patient. *British Medical Journal,* 1970, 389–393.

Craven, J., & Wald, F. Hospice care for dying patients. *American Journal of Nursing,* 1975, *75,* 1821.

Cutter, F. *Coming to terms with death: How to face the inevitable with wisdom and dignity.* Chicago: Nelson-Hall, 1974.

Dana, B. The integration of medicine and other community services. In *Catastrophic illness: Impact on families, challenge to the professions,* symposium proceedings. New York: Cancer Care, Inc. of the National Cancer Foundation, 1966.

Death Education, an international quarterly on pedagogy, counseling, and care, started in 1977 and available from Hemisphere Publishing Corp, 1025 Vermont Ave. N.W., Washington, D.C. 20005.

Death with dignity—at home. *The Washington Post,* November 16, 1975, p. A10.

Deitz, J. H. Rehabilitation of the cancer patient. *Medical Clinics of North America,* 1969, *53,* 3.

Department of Health, Education and Welfare. *A guide for promoting home health services.* Washington, D.C.: U. S. Government Printing Office, 1971.

Department of Health, Education and Welfare, Office of the Assistant Secretary for Planning and Evaluation. *Catastrophic illnesses and costs.* Washington, D.C., U. S. Government Printing Office, 1971.

Department of Health, Education and Welfare, Social Security Administration. Private health insurance in 1970. *Social Security Bulletin,* 1972, *35,* 2.

Department of Health, Education and Welfare Vital Health Statistics. *Mortality trends for leading causes of death, United States.* Series 20, Number 16, see especially pp. 1–7, 1950–1969.

Desich, A. The nurse's most difficult function: terminal care. *R. N.,* 1964, *27,* 45–48.

Dickstein, L. S., & Blatt, S. J. Death concern, futurity, and anticipation. *Journal of Consulting Psychology,* 1966, *30,* 11–17.

Diggory, J. C., & Rothman, D. A. Values destroyed by death. *Journal of Abnormal and Social Psychology, 63,* 205–209.

Dobihal, E. Talk or terminal care? *Connecticut Medicine,* 1974, *38,* 365.

Drellich, M. G., & Sutherland, A. M. The psychological impact of cancer and cancer surgery: VI. Adaptation to hysterectomy. *Cancer,* 1956, *9,* 1120.

Duff, R. S., & Hollingshead, A. B. *Sickness and society.* New York: Harper and Row, 1968, p. 307.

Dyk, R. B., & Sutherland, A. M. Adaptation of the spouse and family members to the colostomy patient. *Cancer,* 1956, *9,* 123–138.

Eaton, J. W. The art of aging and dying. *The Gerontologist,* 1964, *4,* 94–100.

Editorial. Understanding pain. *Lancet,* 1971, *1,* 1284.

Ehrenreich, B. & Ehrenreich, J. *The American health empire: Power, profits and politics.* New York: Random House, 1970.

Eissler, K. R. *The psychiatrist and the dying patient.* New York: International Universities Press, 1969.

Ekblom, B. Significance of socio-psychological factors with regard to risk of death among elderly persons. *Acta Psychiatrica Scandinavica,* 1963, *39,* 627–633.

Engel, G. Grief and grieving. *American Journal of Nursing,* 1964, *64,* 93–98.

Engel, G. V. Professional autonomy and bureaucratic organization. *Administrative Science Quarterly,* 1970, *15,* 12–21.

Evans, J. *Living with a man who is dying.* New York: Taplinger, 1971.

Exton-Smith, A. N. Terminal illness in the aged. *Lancet,* 1961, *2,* 205.

Fassler, J. *My grandpa died today.* New York: Behavioral Publications, 1971.

Feder, S. L. Attitudes of patients with advanced malignancy. *Symposium of the Group for the Advancement of Psychiatry,* 1965, *5,* 614–622.

Feifel, H. Attitudes of mentally ill patients towards death. *Journal of Nervous and Mental Diseases,* 1955, *122,* 375.

Feifel, H. (Ed.). *New meanings of death.* New York: McGraw-Hill, 1977.

Feifel, H. Older persons look at death. *Geriatrics* 1956, *11,* 127.

Feifel. H. (Ed.). *The meaning of death.* New York: McGraw-Hill, 1959.

Feifel, H. The function of attitudes toward death. In *Death and dying: Attitudes of Patient and Doctor,* symposium no. 11, New York: Group for the Advancement of Psychiatry, 1965.

Feifel, H., Hanson, S., Jones, R., & Edwards, L. Physicians consider death. proceedings of the 75th Annual Convention of the American Psychological Association. 1967, *2,* 201–202.

Fein, R. The case for national health insurance. *Saturday Review,* 1970, *53,* 27–29.

Fink, R. Financing outpatient mental health care through psychiatric insurance. *Mental Hygiene, 55,* 143–150.

Fitts, W. T. Jr., & Ravdin, I. S. What Philadelphia physicians tell patients with cancer. *Journal of the American Medical Association,* 1953, *153,* 901–904.

Folck, M. M., & Nie, P. J. Nursing students learn to face death. *Nursing Outlook,* 1959, *7,* 510–513.

Foster, Z. P. How social work can influence hospital management of fatal illness. *Social Work,* 1965, *10,* 4.

Foundation of Thanatology. *Bereavement and illness.* New York: H. S. Publishing Corp., 1973.

Friedman, S. B. Behavioral observations on parents anticipating the death of a child. *Pediatrics,* 1963, *32,* 610.

Freidson, E. *Professional dominance.* New York: Atherton, 1970.

From a Special Correspondent. Vocational training for general practice, 1. A district hospitals scheme: Ipswich. *British Medical Journal,* 1971, *2,* 704.

Fulton, R. *Death and identity.* New York: Wiley, 1965.

Fulton, R. *A bibliography on death, grief and bereavement, 1845–1973,* (3rd ed.). Minneapolis: University of Minnesota Center for Death Education and Research, 1973.

Furman, E. *A child's parent dies.* New Haven: Yale University Press, 1974.

Garner, H. H. *Psychosomatic management of the patient with malignancy.* Springfield, Ill.: Charles C Thomas, 1966.

Gavey, C. J. *The management of the hopeless case.* London: H. K. Lewis, 1952.

Geiger, H. J. Challenge to the professions. In *Catastrophic illness: impact on families. Challenge to the professions,* symposium proceedings. New York: Cancer Care, Inc. of the National Cancer Foundation, 1966.

Gemwill, P. F. *Britain's search for health: The first decade of the national health service.*

Gerle, B., Lunden, G., & Sanblom, P. The patient with inoperable cancer from the psychiatric and social standpoints. A study of 101 cases. *Cancer,* 1960, *13,* 1206–1217.

Glaser, B., & Strauss, A. *Awareness of dying.* Aldive, 1965.

Glaser, B. G. The social loss of dying patients. *American Journal of Nursing,* 1964, 119–121.

Glaser, B. G. Disclosure of terminal illness. *Journal of Health and Human Behavior,* 1966, *7,* 83–91.

Glaser, B. G., & Strauss, A. L. Dying on time. *Transaction,* 1965, *2,* 27–31.

Glaser, B. G., & Strauss, A. L. *Time for dying.* Chicago: Aldine 1968.

Goldberg, et al. (Eds.). *Medical care of the dying patient.* New York: H. S. Publishing, 1973.

Goldfarb, A. L. The psychiatric aspects of integrated services for the terminal ill patient and his family. Report of a symposium on terminal illness. New York: Cancer Care, Inc. of the National Cancer Foundation, 1956.

Goldfarb, D., & Poe, F. T. Meeting needs in terminal illness: Care at home or care outside the home. In *Symposium proceedings, a constructive approach to terminal illness.* New York: Cancer Care, Inc. of the National Cancer Foundation, 1958.

Gorer, G. *Exploring English character.* London: Cresset Press, 1965.

Gorer, G. *Death, grief and mourning.* New York: Doubleday, 1965.

Green, B., et al. *Death education: Preparation for living.* Cambridge, Massachusetts: Schenkman, 1971.

Greene, W. A. What the cancer patient should be told about his diagnosis and prognosis. In *The physician and the total care of the cancer patient.* New York: The American Cancer Society, 1962, 69–73.

Grollman, E. A. (Ed.). *Concerning death: A practical guide for the living.* Boston: Beacon Press, 1974.

Grollman, E. A. *Explaining death to children.* Boston: Beacon Press, 1967.

Grosser, G. H., Wechsler, H., & Greenblatt, M. (Eds.). *The threat of impending disaster.* Cambridge, Mass: MIT Press, 1964.

Group for the Advancement of Psychiatry, Death and Dying: Attitudes of patient and doctor, symposium no. 11,5,9, 1965.

Gunther, J. *Death be not proud.* New York: Harper, 1950.

Hackett, T. P. How to help the dying patient. *Medical Economics,* 1966, *43,* 2–6.

Hackett, R. P., & Weisman, A. Treatment of the dying. In J. Masserman (Ed.), *Current psychiatric therapies.* New York: Grune & Stratton, pp. 121–126.

Hamovitch, M. B. *The parent and the fatally ill child.* Duarte, Calif.: City of Hope Medical Center, 1964.

Harris, E. G. The physician, the clergyman, and the patient in terminal illness. *Pennsylvania Medical Journal,* 1951, *54,* 541–545.

Henderson, L. J. Physician and patient as a social system. *New England Journal of Medicine,* 1935, *212,* 819.

Hinton, J. M. The physical and mental distress of the dying. *Quarterly Journal of Medicine,* 1963, *32,* 1.

Hinton, J. M. Problems of the dying. *Journal of Chronic Diseases,* 1964, *17,* 201–205.

Hinton, J. M. Talking with people about to die. *British Medical Journal,* 1974, 225–227.

Hodgins, E. *Episode.* New York: Athenaeum, 1964.

Holden, C. Hospices: For the dying, relief from pain and fear. *Science,* 1976, *193,* 389.

Hollender, M. H. The patient with carcinoma. *The psychology of medical practice.* Philadelphia: Saunder, 1958, pp. 89–115.

Horder, T. J. Signs and symptoms of impending death. *Practitioner,* 1948, *161,* 73–75.

Howard, A., & Scott, R. A. Cultural values and attitudes toward death. *Journal of Existentialism,* 1965, *6,* 161–174.

Hughes, H. L. G. *Peace at last.* London: Calouste Gulbenkian Foundation, 1960.

Institute of Medicine of Chicago. *Terminal care of cancer patients.* Chicago: Institute of Medicine, 1961.

Isaacs, B. Changes in the demand for geriatric care. *Gerontological Clinics,* 1970, *12,* 257–266.

Jackson, E. N. *For the living.* Des Moines: Channel Press, 1963.

Jackson, E. N. Resources for facing new horizons. In *Catastrophic illness: impact on families, challenge to the professions,* symposium proceedings. New York: Cancer Care, Inc. of the National Cancer Foundation, 1966.

Jackson, R. R., Spencer, W. A., Vallbona, C., Harrison, G. M., & Hoff, H. E. Principles of organization for the care of the severely disabled. *Archives of Physical Medicine and Rehabilitation,* 1961, *42,* 526.

Kalish, R. A. Some variables in death attitudes. *Journal of Social Psychology,* 1963, *59,* 137–145.

Kalish, R. A. The aged and the dying process: The inevitable decisions. *Journal of Social Issues,* 1965, *21,* 87–96.

Kalish, R. A., A continuum of subjectively perceived death. *The Gerontologist,* 1966, *6,* 73–76.

Kalish, R. A. Social distance and the dying. *Community Mental Health Journal,* 1966, *2,* 152–155.

Kalish, R. A. Life and death: Dividing the indivisable. *Social Science and Medicine,* 1968, *2,* 249–259.

Kastenbaum, R. (Ed.). *Death and dying.* (40 Vols.). New York, Arno, 1977.

Kastenbaum, R. *Death, society and human behavior.* St. Louis, Mosby, 1977.

Kastenbaum, R., & Avery, W. *The psychological autopsy.* New York: Human Sciences Press, 1968.

Kastenbaum, R. The reluctant therapist. *Geriatrics,* 1963, *18,* 296–301.

Kastenbaum, R. The realm of death: An emerging area in psychological research. *Journal of Human Relations,* 1965, *13,* 538–552.

Kastenbaum, R., & Aisenberg, R. *The psychology of death.* New York: Springer Publishing, 1972.

Kaufmann, W. Death in the fairy tale. *Diseases of the Nervous System,* 1968, *28,* 462–468.

Keeler, W. R. Children's reaction to the death of a parent. In P. H. Hoch, & J. Zubin (Eds.) Depression proceedings of the 42nd Annual Meeting of the American Psychopathological Association. New York: Grune & Stratton, 1954, pp. 109–120.

Kellett, T. E. The dying patient and the hospital: An attitude sampling. *Hospital Administration,* 1965, *10,* 26–37.

Kelly, W. D., & Friesen, S. R. Do cancer patients want to be told? *Surgery,* 1950, *27,* 822–26.

Kennedy, N., Leslie, R. C., & Wahl, C. W. *Helping the dying patient and his family, pamphlet 336.* New York: National Association of Social Workers, 1960.

Kennedy, N., Leslie, R. C., & Wahl, C. W. *Helping the dying patient and his family, pamphlet 336.* New York: National Association of Social Workers, 1960.

Kennedy, E. M. *In critical condition.* New York: Simon and Schuster, 1972.

Knudson, A. G., & Natterson, J. M. Participation of parents in the hospital care of fatally ill children. *Pediatrics,* 1960, *26,* 482–490.

Kohn, J. Hospice movement provides humane alternative for terminally ill patients. *Modern Healthcare,* 1976, 26.

Krant, M. J. The question of irradiation therapy in lung cancer. *Journal of The American Medical Association,* 1966, *195,* 177–181.

Krant, M. J. *Dying and dignity—The meaning and control of a personal death.* Springfield, Ill.: Charles C Thomas.

Kraus, A. S., & Lilifenfield, A. M. Some epidemiological aspects of the high mortality rate in the young widowed group. *Journal of Chronic Diseases,* 1959, *10,* 207–217.

Kron, J. Designing a better place to die. *New York,* March 1, 1976, p. 43.

Kubler-Ross, E. The dying patient as teacher: An experiment and an experience. *The Chicago Theological Seminary Register,* 1966, *57,* 3.

Kubler-Ross, E. Psychotherapy with the least expected. *Rehabilitation Literature,* 1968, *29,* 73–76.

Kubler-Ross, E. *On death and dying.* New York: Macmillan, 1970.

Kubler-Ross, E. The care of the dying—Whose job is it? *Psychosomatic Medicine,* 1970, *1,* 103–107.

Kubler-Ross, E. *The dying patient's point of view. The dying patient.* New York: Russell Sage Foundation, 1970.

Kubler-Ross, E. *Death—the final stage of growth.* New York: Macmillan, 1975.

Kutner, B. Terminal illness and death in socio-cultural perspective. *A constructive approach to terminal illness,* symposium proceedings. New York: Cancer Care, Inc. of the National Cancer Foundation, 1958.

Kutscher, A. H., & Kutscher, A. H., Jr. *A bibliography of books on death, bereavement, loss and grief: 1935–1968.* New York: Health Sciences.

Kutscher, A. H., & Kutscher, A. H., Jr. *Supplement I. A bibliography of books of death, bereavement, loss and grief: 1968–.*

Kutscher, M. et al. *A comprehensive bibliography of the thanatology literature.* MSS Information Corporation, 1975. A large bibliography under the copyright of the Foundation of Thanatology, with 4,844 references.

Lack, S., & Lamterton, R. (Eds.). *The hour of our death.* London: Geoffrey Chapman, 1974.

Lamerton, R. *Care of the dying.* London: Priory Press, Ltd., 1973.

Lampedusa, G. di. *The leopard.* Translated by Archibald Colquhoun. New York: Pantheon Books, 1960.

Langer, M. *Learning to live as a widow.* New York: Julian Messner, 1957.

Lasagna, L. *Life, death and the doctor.* New York: Knopf, 1968.

Lawrence, M. *Interrupted melody; The story of my life.* New York: Appleton-Century-Crofts, 1969.

Laycock, J. D. Pain relieving drugs. *St. Thomas's Hospital Gazette,* 1959, *5.*

Legislative Memorandum, Published by the Community Service Society of New York, Department of Public Affairs, New York.

Leonard, K. Frequency of the various forms of neurosis in different time periods. *Psychiatry, Neurology, Medical Psychology,* 1971, *23,* 29–137.

LeShan, L. L. The world of the patient in severe pain of long duration. *The Journal of Chronic Diseases,* 1964, *17,* 119–126.

LeShan, L. L. Psychotherapy with the dying. In *Care of the Dying* symposium of the New York Academy of Sciences. New York: 1969.

LeShan, L. L., & LeShan, E. Psychotherapy and the patient with a limited life span. *Psychiatry,* 1961, *24,* 318–23.

LeShan, L. L., Jackson, E., Bowers, M., & Knight, J. *Counseling the dying patient.* Camden, N.J.: Thomas Nelson and Sons, 1965.

Lester, D. Experimental and correlational studies of the fear of death. *Psychological Bulletin,* 1967, *67,* 27–36.

Leveton, A. Time, death and the ego-chill. *Journal of Existentialism,* 1965, *6,* 69–80.

Lifton, R. J., & Olson, E. *Living and dying.* New York: Praeger, 1975.

Lindemann, E. Symptomatology and management of acute grief. *American Journal of Psychiatry* 1944, *101,* 141–48.

Lipman, A., & Marden, P. W. Preparation for death in old age. *Journal of Gerontology,* 1966, *21,* 426–431.

Lowry, R. J. *Male-female differences in attitudes toward death.* (Ph.D. Dissertation). Waltham, Massachusetts: Brandeis University, 1965.

MacLaurin, H. In the hour of their going forth. *Social Casework,* 1959, *40,* 136–141.

Mann, T. *The magic mountain.* Translated by H. T. Lowe-Porter. New York: Modern Library, 1932.

Mannes, M. *Last rights, a case for the good death.* New York: Morrow, 1973.

Marks, E. *Simone de Beauvoir: Encounters with death.* New Brunswick, N.J.: Rutgers University Press, 1973.

Marshall, C. *A man called Peter.* New York: McGraw-Hill, 1951.

Marris, P. *Widows and their families.* London: Routledge and Kegan, Paul 1958.

Marston, R. Q. The regional medical programs for heart, cancer, stroke and related diseases. In *Catastrophic illness: Impact on families, challenge to the professions,* symposium proceedings. New York: Cancer Care, Inc., of the National Cancer Foundation, 1966.

Martin, D., & Wrightsman, L. S. The relationship between religious behavior and concern about death. *Journal of Social Psychology,* 1965, *65,* 317–323.

Masserman, J. (Ed.). *Current psychiatric therapies, 1.* New York: Grune & Stratton, 1961.

Matterson, J. M., & Knudson, A. G. Observations concerning fear of death in fatally ill children and their mothers. *Psychosomatic Medicine,* 1960, *22,* 456–465.

McCormack, P. Helping hands, hearts for terminally ill. *The Hartford Times,* March 14, 1976.

McCullers, C. *Clock without hands.* Boston: Houghton-Mifflin, 1961.

McDonald, B. *Who, me?* Philadelphia: J. B. Lippincott, 1959.

McDonald, M. Helping children to understand health: An experience with death in a nursery school. *Journal of Nursery School Education,* 1963, *19,* 19–25.

McMahon, B., Pugh, F. F., & Ibsen, J. *Epidemiological methods.* Boston: Little, Brown, 1960.

McNulty, B. J. St. Christopher's outpatients. *American Journal of Nursing,* 1971, *71,* 23–28.

Meany, G. National health insurance: Labor's number one legislative goal. *Vital Speeches,* 1970, *37,* 14–16.

Miller, M. Decision making in the death process in the ill aged. *Geriatrics,* 1971, 105–116.

Nagler, J. H. Care of the terminal cancer patient. *Journal of the American Geriatrics Society,* 1956, *4,* 699–707.

National Cancer Survey. London: 1952.

National Council for Homemaker-Home Health Aide Services, Inc. *An agenda for action, forum report.* New York, 1972.

National Council for Homemaker-Home Health Aide Services, Inc. *Resource book on financing homemaker-home health aide services.* New York, 1972.

Neale, R. E. *The art of dying.* New York: Harper, 1973.

Nevinny, H. B., Hall, T. C., & Krant, M. J. Comparison of Methotrexate (NSC 740) and Testosterone (NSC 9166) in the treatment of breast cancer. *The Journal of Clinical Pharmacology,* 1968, *8,* 128–9.

Newman, E. *Death psychology and the new ethic.* New York: Harper, 1973.

Nielson, M., & Beggs, H. *Home aide service and the aged: A controlled study.* Springfield, Virginia, U.S. Department of Commerce, National Technical Information Service, 1972.

1976 NIH Almanac (DHEW No. NIH 76–5) pp. 1–21.

Norton, J. Treatment of a dying patient. *Psychoanalytic Study of the Child,* 1963, *18,* 541–60.

Oken, D. What to tell cancer patients. *Journal of the American Medical Association,* 1961, *175,* 1120.

Osler, W. *Science and immortality.* London: Constable, 1906.

Parkes, C. M. Effects of bereavement: on physical and mental—Study of the medical records of widows. *British Medical Journal,* 1964, *2,* 274–279.

Parkes, C. M. Recent bereavement as a cause of mental illness. *British Medical Journal of Psychiatry,* 1964, *116,* 198.

Parkes, C. M. Bereavement and mental illness, pt. 1, a clinical study of the grief of bereaved psychiatric patients; pt. 2, classification of bereavement reactions. *British Journal of Medical Psychology*, 1965, *38*, 1.

Parkes, C. M. The first year of bereavement. *Psychiatry*, 1971, *33*, 444.

Parkes, C. M. Accuracy of predictions of survival in later stages of cancer. *British Medical Journal*, 1972, 29.

Parkes, C. M. Components of the reaction to loss of a limb, spouse or home. *Journal of Psychosomatic Research*, 1972, *16*, 383–349.

Parkes, C. M. The first year of bereavement: A longitudinal study of the reaction of London widows to the death of their husbands. *Psychiatry*, 1971, *23*, 444.

Patry, F. L. A psychiatric evaluation of communicating with the dying. *Diseases of the Nervous System*, 1965, *26*, 715–718.

Payne, E. C. Jr. The physician and his patient who is dying. In S. Levin, & R. J. Kahana (Eds.), *Psychodynamic studies on aging: Creativity, reminiscing and dying.* New York, International Universities Press, 1967, 111–163.

Payne, E. C., & Krant, M. J. The psychological aspects of advanced cancer. *Journal of the American Medical Association*, 1969, *210*, 1236.

Pearson, L. *Death and dying: Current issues in the treatment of the dying patient.* Cleveland, Ohio: Press of Case Western Reserve University, 1969.

Peniston, D. H. The importance of 'death education' in family life. *Family Life Coordinator*, 1967, *11*, 15–18.

Perspectives in long-term care. Chicago: American Medical Association.

Pettengill, D. W. Writing the prescription for health care. *Harvard Business Review*, 1971, *49*, 37–43.

Pollock, G. H. Mourning and adaptation. *International Journal of Psychoanalysis*, 1961, *42*, 341–361.

Poteet, G. H. *Death and dying, a bibliography* (1950–1974). Whitson Publishing, 1976. Contains a large number of references to journal articles on the psychology of death.

Quint, J. C. *The nurse and the dying patient.* New York: Macmillan, 1967.

Quint, J. C. The dying patient: A difficult nursing problem. *Nursing Clinics of North America*, 1967, *2*, 763–773.

Quint, J. C. The impact of mastectomy. *American Journal of Nursing*, 1963, *63*, 88–97.

Rees, W. D., & Lutkins, S. G. Mortality of bereavement. *British Medical Journal*, 1967, *4*, 13.

Research and related programs of the National Cancer Institute. Public Health Service Publication No. 458-A, revised in 1969, p. 10.

Rice, D. Estimating the cost of illness. Publication #947–6, Washington, D.C.: U.S. Public Health Service.

Richmond, J. B., & Waisman, H. A. Psychologic aspects of management of children with malignant diseases. *American Journal of Diseases of Children*, 1955, *89*, 42–47.

Rochlin, G. *Griefs and discontents.* Boston: Little, Brown, 1965.

Rolansky, J. D. (Ed.). *The end of life.* New York: Fleet Press Corporation, 1973.

Rossman, I. Suitability of home care for the cancer patient. *Geriatrics*, 1956, *2*, 407–12.

Rossman, I. Treatment of cancer on a home care program. *The Journal of the American Medical Association*, 1954, *156*, 827.

Rossman, I. Reduction of anxiety in a home care setting. *The Journal of Chronic Diseases*, 1956, *4*, 527–534.

Rossman, I., Rudnick, B., & Clarke, M. Total rehabilitation in home care setting. *New York State Medical Journal*, 1962, *62*, 1215–1219.

Rossman, I., Cherkasky, M., & Rogatz, P. *Guide to organized home care.* Chicago: Hospital Research and Education Trust, 1960.

Rossman, I., & Kissick, W. L. Home Care and the cancer patient. *The physician and the total care of the cancer patient.* New York: Macmillan, 1967.

Rothenberg, A. Psychological problems in terminal cancer. *Cancer*, 1961, *14*, 1663–1673.

Ruark, R. *The honey badger.* New York: McGraw-Hill, 1965.

Ruitenbeek, H. M. *The interpretation of death.* New York: J. Aronson, 1973.

Russel, H. *Victory in my hands.* New York: Creative Age Press, 1949.

Russell, W. R. Discussion on the treatment of intractable pain. *Proceedings of the Royal Society of Medicine,* 1959, *52,* 983.

Saunders, C. A patient. *Nursing Times,* 1961.

Saunders, C. *Care of the dying.* London: Macmillan, 1959.

Saunders, C. The treatment of intractable pain in terminal cancer. *Proceedings of the Royal Society of Medicine,* 1963, *56,* 191–197.

Saunders, C. Watch with me. *Nursing Times,* 1965.

Saunders, C. The management of fatal illness in childhood. *Proceedings of the Royal Society of Medicine,* 1969, *62,* 550–53.

Saunders, C. Death and responsibility: A medical director's view. *Psychiatric Opinion,* 1966, *3,* 28–34.

Saunders, C. The management of terminal illness. *Hospital Medicine,* 1966, pt. 1, 225–228; pt. 2, 317–320; pt. 3, 433–436.

Saunders, C. The last stages of life. *American Journal of Nursing,* 1965, *65,* 70–75.

Saunders, C. The need for in-patient care for the patient with terminal cancer. *Middlesex Hospital Journal,* 1973, *72,* 3.

Saunders, C. Training for the practice of clinical gerontology: The role of social medicine. *Interdiscipl. Topics Geront.,* 1970, *5,* 72–78.

Schlesinger, L. E. Disruption in the personal-social system resulting from traumatic disability. *Journal of Health and Human Behavior,* 1965, *6,* 91–99.

Schmale, A. H., & Iker, H. P. The effect of hopelessness and the development of cancer: I. Identification of uterine cervical cancer in women with atypical cytology. *Psychosomatic Medicine,* 1966, *28,* 714–721.

Schoenberg, B. et al. *Anticipatory grief.* New York: Columbia University Press, 1974.

Schoenberg, B., Car, A. C., Peretz, D., & Kutscher, A. H. *Loss and grief: psychological management in medical practice.* New York: Columbia University Press, 1970.

Schoenrich, E. H. Comprehensive care for the catastrophically ill. In *Catastrophic illness in the seventies: critical issues and complex decisions,* symposium proceedings. New York: Cancer Care, Inc. of the National Cancer Foundation, 1971.

Scofield, P. B. Analgesics in terminal disease. *British Medical Journal,* 1971, *2,* 773.

Schur, M. The problem of death in Freud's writings and life. *Journal of Psychiatry,* 1965, *34,* 144–147.

Sechzer, P. H. Objective measurement of pain. *Anesthesiology, 1968, 29,* 209.

Sechzer, P. H. Studies in pain with the analgesic demand system. 44th Congress of the International Anesthesia Research Society. Palm Springs, Calif.: 1970.

Sheldon, A., Ryser, C. P., & Krant, M. J. An integrated family orientated cancer care program: The report of a pilot project in the socio-emotional management of chronic disease. *The Journal of Chronic Diseases,* 1970, *22,* 743–55.

Sheldon, J. H. *The social medicine of old age.* London: Oxford University Press, 1948.

Shepard, M. *Someone you love is dying: A guide for helping and coping.* New York: Harmony Books, 1975.

Shibles, W. *Death: An interdisciplinary analysis.* Whitewater, Wisc.: Language Press, 1974.

Shneidman, E. S. *Death and the college student.* New York: Behavioral Publications, 1972.

Silver, G. A. Insurance is not enough. *The Nation,* 1970, *210,* 680–683.

Siegel, D., & Stein, F. The place of the medical social worker in the home care of the long-term patient. In a report of an Arden House Conference of the National Foundation for Infantile Paralysis. Harriman, N.Y.: 1953.

Silverman, A. J., Busse, E. W., Barnes, R. H., Thaler, M. B., & Frost, L. L. Physiologic influences on psychic functioning in elderly people. *Geriatrics,* 1953, *8,* 370–76.

Snow, C. P. *The light and the dark.* New York: Charles Scribner's Sons, 1961.

Somers, H. M., & Ramsey, A. *Doctors, patients, and health insurance: The organization and financing of medical care.* Washington, D.C.: The Brookings Institution, 1961.

Spilka, B., Pellegrini, R., & Bailey, K. Religion, American values and death responsibilities. *Sociological Symposium,* 1968, 57–66.

Sprott, N. A. Dying of cancer. *Medical Press and Circular,* 1949, *221,* 197.

Standard, S., & Nathan, H. *Should the patient know the truth?* New York: Springer, 1955.

State of New York, Department of Labor, Report to Governor Nelson A. Rockefeller of the Special Task Force to Study Catastrophic Health Insurance. 4 Vols. Albany, New York.

Stehlin, J. S. Jr., & Beach, K. H. Psychological aspects of cancer therapy, A surgeon's viewpoint. *Journal of the American Medical Association,* 1966, *197,* 100.

Stein, A., & Susser, M. W. Widowhood and mental illness. *British Journal of Preventative and Social Medicine,* 1969, *23,* 106.

Stern, K., Williams, G. M., Prados, M. Grief reactions in later life. *American Journal of Psychiatry,* 1951–52, *108,* 289–94.

Strauss, A. Family and staff weeks and days of terminal illness. *Annals of N.Y. Academy of Science,* 1969, *164,* 587.

Strauss, A., Glaser, B., & Quint, J. The nonaccountability of terminal care hospitals. *Journal of the American Hospital Association,* 1964, *38,* 73–87.

Strauss, A. L., & Glaser, B. G. *Anguish.* Mill Valley, CA: Sociology Press, 1970.

Sudnow, D. *Passing on.* Englewood Cliffs, N.J.: Prentice-Hall, 1967.

Sutherland, A. M. The psychological impact of cancer and its therapy. *Medical Clinics of North America,* 1956, *40,* 705–720.

Sutherland, A. M., Orback, C. E., Dyk, R. B., & Bard, M. The psychological impact of cancer surgery, I. Adaptation to the dry colostomy. *Cancer,* 1952, *5,* 857.

Swenson, W. M. Attitudes toward death among the aged, *Minnesota Medicine,* 1959, *42,* 399.

Tanner, J. M. (Ed.). *Stress and psychiatric disorder.* Oxford: Blackwell Scientific Publications, 1960.

1975 revised edition of The National Cancer Institute, published by the U.S. Department of Health, Education and Welfare (No. NIH 76–792).

Thomas, A. G. Psychosocial aspects of cancer: Typical patient and family attitudes. *Public Health Reports,* 1952, *67,* 10.

Thomas, A. G. New approaches to old problems. *Medical Social Work,* 1955, *4,* 1.

Tolstoy, L. *The death of Ivan Ilytch.* New York: New American Library, 1960.

Trager, B. Home Health Services in the United States: A Report Prepared for the Committee on Aging of the U.S. Senate. Washington, D.C.: U.S. Government Printing Office, 1972.

Troup, S. B., et al. (Eds.). *Patient, death, and the family.* New York: Scribner, 1974.

Tucker, M. A. Effects of heavy expenditures on low-income families. *Public Health Reports,* 1970, *85,* 419–425.

Turnbull, Intractable pain. *Proceedings of the Royal Society of Medicine,* 1954, *47,* 155.

Verwoerdt, A., & Elmore, J. L. Psychological reactions in fatal illness. I. The prospect of impending death. *Journal of the American Geriatrics Society,* 1967, *15,* 9–19.

Waechter, E. H. Children's awareness of fatal illness. *American Journal of Nursing,* 1971, *71,* 1168.

Wagner, B. Teaching students to work with the dying. *American Journal of Nursing,* 1964, *64,* 178–131.

Wahl, C. W. The fear of death. *Bulletin of the Menninger Clinic,* 1958, *22,* 214.

Washington Bulletin, published bi-monthly by Social Legislation Information Service, Inc., Washington, D.C.

Washington Report on Medicine and Health, published weekly, McGraw-Hill, Inc., Washington, D.C.

Waxenberg, S. Hopeful aspects of social worker communication with cancer patients. Memorial Hospital for Cancer and Allied Disease, New York.

Weisman, A. *On dying and denying:* A psychiatric study of terminality. New York: Human Sciences Press, 1972.

Westberg, G. E. *Good grief.* Philadelphia: Fortress Press, 1962.

Whitehead, A. *In the service of old age: The welfare of psychogeriatric patients.* Pelican, p. 59.

Wilkes, E. Cancer outside hospital. *Lancet,* 1964, *1,* 1379.

Wilkes, E. Terminal cancer at home. *Lancet,* 1965, *1,* 799.

Williams, R. L., & Cole, S. Religiosity, generalized anxiety, and apprehension concerning death. *Journal of Social Psychology,* 1968, *75,* 111–117.

Wolff, K. Helping elderly patients face the fear of death. *Hospital and Community Psychiatry,* 1967, *18,* 142–144.

Worcester, A. *Care of the aged, the dying and the dead.* Springfield, Ill: Charles C Thomas, 1935.

Young, M., Benjamin, B., & Wallis, C. *Lancet,* 1963, *2,* 454.

Zaltman, G., Duncan, R., & Holbek, J. Innovations in organization. New York: Wiley and Sons, 1973.

Zinsser, H. *As I remember him.* Boston: Little, Brown, 1964.

Index

Accidental deaths, concern
with, 56
Addiction, fear of, 73
Aderman, David, 47
Admissions, number of, to
St. Christopher's
Hospice, 70, 80
Afterlife, 39, 41
Age of patients
in Hospice, Inc., Home
Care Program, 94
at St. Christopher's
Hospice, 82
Aged, *See* Elderly
Aisenberg, R., 38, 40, 41,
53, 55–57
American Cancer Society,
34–35

American Indians, cancer
data on, 31, 34
Analgesics, *See* Pain
management
Anger, as reaction to
illness, 39, 43, 44
Anorexia, 70, 98–99
Anticholinergic symptoms,
99
Anticipatory grief, 45
Anxiety
of acutely ill children, 39
alleviation of, 99
in health personnel
caring for dying
patients, 49
hospice design and, 103

Autopsy, hospice attitudes toward, 73
Avoidance, of dying patients, 49, 50

Baltimore Cancer Research Center, 141
Bartlett, Dr., 130
Belgian Gheel community, 12
Benzodiazepines, 99
Bereaved
children, 38–39
follow-up visits to, 75
as hospice staff members, 63, 95–96
and hospices in hospitals, 135
needs of, 58
professional management of, 45, 52–53
See also Bereavement
Bereavement, 44–45
signs and symptoms of, 52
stages of, 45
Black people, mortality rates for, compared with whites, 23
See also Race
Blue Cross, 100, 108, 109
Breathlessness, 70
"Brompton's cocktail," 71

Budgets
estimated, for Strong Hospice, 126–127
of Hospice, Inc., 109
of National Institutes of Health, 142, 143, 145–149, 155–157
Burke, Lawrence, 158–159, 163

Calvary Hospital, New York City, 135–136
Cancer
as cause of death, 23, 117
cure rates for, 34–35
delay in seeking treatment for, 42
as potential hospice care category, 30
race and sex associated with incidence of, 30–34
race and site of, 31
type of, factors influencing, 30
See also Cancer death; Cancer patients
Cancer Center, Rochester, New York, 114
Cancer death
methods of coping with, 45–46

[Cancer death]
by race and sex from
1950–1973, 32–33
research on, 34–35
site of, 91
Cancer patients
admission to Hospice
Home Care Program,
93
children, 39
hospices and, 28
length of stay at St.
Christopher's, 92
in nursing homes, 16–17
pain and, 98
primary site of tumors
in, 81
refusal of further
treatment by, 29
Carcinogens, cancer rates
by geographic regions
and, 34
Cardiovascular-renal
conditions, as cause of
death, 23
Case study method of
hospice evaluation,
67
Chan, Lo Yi, 64, 102, 105
Chapel, in hospice, 79
Chemotherapy, 159
Children
bereaved, 39
Hospice, Inc., and, 105

[Children]
and life of hospice, 64,
74
response to death, 38–40
Chinese-Americans, cancer
death data on, 31, 34
Clergy, counseling for
dying by, 17, 54
Clinic, at St. Christopher's,
75–76
Cocaine, in pain
management, 71
Commonwealth Fund, 89,
90
Community, institutional
lag in response to
hospice movement
and, 166
Community education,
support for hospices
and, 89, 108
Community health care
planners, evaluation of
hospices and, 15–18
Community resources
in assessment of Strong
Hospice plan, 119
inadequacies of, 16–18
Connecticut Commission
on Hospitals and
Health Care, 107–108
Connecticut Medicine,
86–87
Constipation, 98

Convalescent homes, *See* Nursing and convalescent homes

Coping mechanisms, 45–47 selection of, 41–52

Counseling for dying patients and families, inadequacies of, 17

Craven, Joan, 97

Cultural factors, death process and, 55–57

Davenport-Hatch Foundations, 116

Day-care in hospices, 64, 78, 105

Death
acceptance of, 17
American view of, 55–57
changes in causes of, 20, 21, 23–24, 26–27
parental reaction to, 39
prevention of, as function of medical career, 48
as taboo topic, 49
of widowers, 44–45
See also Dying children; Dying people; Dying in United States; Fear of death; Individual responses to death; Institutional responses to death

"Death system," culture and, 55–57

Denial, 30, 54

Department of Health, Education and Welfare, 18

Dependency, as reaction to death, 42

Depression, 46, 47

Developmental stage, selection of coping mechanisms and, 41–42

Dexamethasone, 72

Diamorphine, 71

Diarrhea, 98

Discharges, at St. Christopher's, 80

Dobihal, Reverend Edward, 13, 86, 88

Domiciliary Service, St. Christopher's, 69, 70, 75–75

Draper's Wing, St. Christopher's, 79

Drug therapy, *See* Pain management; Polypharmacy

Dubrey, Sister Rita Jean, 53

Duff, Raymong, 54–55

Dunn, Sister Mary Kaye, 97

Dying children, 28–30

[Dying children]
excluded from Strong
Hospice plan, 119–120
information from
pediatricians to parents
of, 48
needs of, 58
Dying people
attitudes of health care
professionals to, 17,
49, 50–51, 117–118
changing awareness in,
47
effect of admission to
hospice on, 70–71
emphasis on medical care
of, 19–20
families of, *see* Families
goals in management of,
49
historical attitudes
toward, 12–13
in hospices, 12
in hospitals, 16, 114
"ideal" behavior of,
50–51, 52
interaction among,
64
literature on, 19–20
needs of, 14–18, 57–58
psychological stages in,
47
site of death of, 91
symptoms of, 98–99

Dying in United States,
37–59
and individual responses
to death, 38–47
and institutional response
to death, 48–57
needs of, 37
and professional
management of
bereaved, 52–53
study of, 37–38

Education
in hospices within
hospitals, 113
at St. Christopher's,
77–78
Elavil, 99
Elderly
Elavil and, 99
increase in numbers of,
20, 25–26, 35–36
and nursing homes,
16–17
residences for, connected
with hospice, 79
End Results in Cancer,
35
England, hospices in, 69
See also St. Christopher's
Hospice
Euthanasia Educational
Council, 116

Evasion, 55
Extinction, fear of, 41

Family(ies)
  continuation of
    relationships with
    hospice staff and
    patients' families,
    78–79
  counseling for, 17
  and design of Hospice
    Inc., inpatient facility,
    104–105
  of dying child, 58–59
  exclusion from intensive
    care units, 15
  at Hospice, Inc., 85,
    92–93
  and hospice care, 12, 18
  and needs assessment for
    Strong Hospice,
    118–119
  role in support of dying
    patient, 53
  at St. Christopher's,
    74–75
  viewing of body by,
    104–105
  visits by, 62
  See also Bereaved;
    Bereavement
Family room, in hospice,
  64

Federal government
  hospice development and,
    18–19, 35–36, 165–166
  national institutes of, 142
  See also National Cancer
    Institute
Fear of death, 19, 40–41,
  42
Flurazepam, 99
Fobihal, Edward F., Jr.,
  86–87
Foundation grants for
  hospices, 90–91, 115
Friends of Hospice, 89
Funding of hospices, 76,
  80, 89, 90, 93, 100,
  106–110, 112, 125,
  128–130, 148-149
Funeral directors, and
  death management, 54

Geographical regions
  cancer incidence by, 30,
    34
  mortality rates and, 23
Glaser, Barbey, 47, 50–51
Goldenberg, Dr. Ira, 86
Gonda, Thomas, 46
Guilt, death and, 39, 43

Health professionals
  management of bereaved
    by, 52–53

[Health professionals]
and needs of dying
patients, 17, 53–55
and polypharmacy,
71–72
training of, 40, 47, 125
Heimlich, Henry, 52
Heroin, *See* Diamorphine
Hollingshead, August,
54–55
Home, cancer deaths in, 91
Home care programs
criteria for, 93–94
proposal at Strong
Hospice, 124
purpose of, 65
See also Home Care
Service
Home Care Service,
Hospice, Inc., 93–98
*Hopeful Side of Cancer,
The,* 34–35
Hospice, Inc., New Haven,
Connecticut, 13,
60–61, 85–110
acceptance by medical
community, 88–89
budget, 109
building committee
plans, 102–104
case histories from,
100–101
compared with St.
Christopher's, 86

[Hospice, Inc.]
decisions on population
serviced by, 91–92
design of, 64, 102–104
exclusion of pediatric
patients, 119–120
founding of, 16, 85,
86–87
funding of, 89, 90, 100,
106–110
hospice movement and,
109–110
influence of St.
Christopher's on,
86–87
licensing of, 107–108
pain control at, 98–100
planning task force,
88–89
principles of care at,
92–93
rates at, 106–107
role as demonstrational
and educational center,
87–88
staff selection at, 63
task forces, 89–90
Hospice Atlanta,
138
Hospice of Buffalo,
New York, 134
Hospice of Marin, Inc.,
Kentfield, California,
137–138

Hospice of Santa Barbara, Inc., 134
Hospice movement, 133–138
and "continuing care" request for Proposals from National Cancer Institute, 159–161
and federal government, *See* National Cancer Institute
institutional lag in response to, 164–167
Hospice staff, 62–63, 68
Hospices, 60–68
admission to, 27–28
and cancer distribution patterns, 35
cause of death and, 20, 27–28
choice of name for, 13
data collection in, 65
definitions of, 12, 13
design of, 63–64, 102–104
and dying children, 28–30
early, 12–13, 60–62
educational role of, 65
evaluation of, 15, 66–67
and families, *See* Families
goals of, 61–62
inadequacies of

[Hospices]
community support system and, 16–18
major components of, 65–66
multidisciplinary approach to, 65
and National Cancer Institute priorities, 148–149, 151–158
and needs of dying patients, 14
outpatient care and, *See* Home care
population necessary to sustain, 133–134
possible effects of, 67–68
program for development of, 88
reasons for opposition to, 19
staffs of, *See* Hospice staff
Hospices within hospitals, 111–114, 135–137
See also Strong Hospital Hospice
Hospitals
attitudes toward anger and fear in, 43
compared with hospices, 73–74
cancer deaths in Connecticut in, 91

[Hospitals]
dying children in, 28–29
families of people dying
in, 53
needs of dying in, 14–15,
16, 114
social class bias in, 54–55
visitors in, 62

Incontinence, 70
Individual responses to
death, 38–47
children and, 38–40
common death reactions,
42–43
and death fear, 40–41
generalized coping
modes, 45–47
and previous personality
factors, 41–42
Infants, dying, 39
Institutional responses to
death, 48–57
cultural factors, 55–57
and management of
bereaved, 52–53
Intensive care units, 14, 15
Intracranial pressure,
polypharmacy and, 72
Issner, Natalie, 38–39

Jackson, Douglas, 44

Japanese-Americans, cancer
incidence in, 31, 34

Kastenbaum, R., 38, 40,
41, 51–52, 53, 55–57
Kohn, Judith, 14
Kubler-Ross, Dr. Elizabeth,
17, 45
Kutscher, Austin, 45, 52

Lack, Dr. Sylvia, 95, 97,
98, 99, 100
Life expectancy, 21
death system and, 55–56
by sex and race, 22, 23

Make Today Count, 128
Marital relationships, and
parents of sick child,
40
Medicaid, 100, 108, 109
Medical care
aggressive, for dying
patients, 114–115
in hospices, 74
reduced mortality rates
and, 23
Medicare, 109
Medication
method of administering,
46

[Medication]
requests for, 72
See also Pain
management
Meditation or screaming
room, 64, 105
Mental health specialists,
dying people and, 54
Monroe County Cancer
and Leukemia
Association (MCCLA),
116–117, 120, 125, 129
Morgue in hospice, 64, 104
Morphine, 99
Mortality data
cancer associated with
race in, 31, 34
changes in, 21
in Connecticut, causes of,
91
for married and
unmarried people, 23
by sex and race, 22, 23
on ward patients, 54–55
Mourning process, before
death of child, 40

Narcotics, *See* Pain
management
National Advisory Cancer
Council, 143–144

National Cancer Act,
139–140
National Cancer Institute
(NCI), 28, 31, 35, 91,
93, 114
approval of grants by,
146
budgets of, 142, 143,
145–149, 151, 155–157
Cancer Control Program
activities of, 149,
150
cancer detection research
of, 141
establishment of,
139–140
and evaluation of
Hospice, Inc., 162
and funding of hospices,
148–149, 151–159
grants of, 143
hospices as threat to,
163–164
organization of, 141–145
priorities of, 145–148
programs of, 150–151
rehabilitation programs
of, 141–142
request for proposals of
(RCP), 159–163
response to hospice
movement, 164–167
and Strong Hospice, 125

National Cancer Program, 140, 143
National Center for Health Statistics, 31
National Health System (Great Britain), 80
  and St. Christopher's, 76–77
National Institute of Health, 18
  budget of, 142
  Clinical Center, 140–141
  research of, 153
Nausea, management of, 69, 71, 98
Nurses
  attitudes toward dying patients, 53–54
  for Home Care Service, 96–97
  at St. Christopher's, 76
  support for hospices from, 117–118
Nursing and convalescent homes, dying patients and, 16–17

Organic brain disease, drugs for, 46
Outpatients, *See* Home care

Pain
  and attitude toward death, 46
  changes in symptoms of, 46–47
  patients with and without problem with, 84
  See also Pain management
Pain management, 46, 71–73
  at Hospice, Inc., 86, 99–101
  at St. Christopher's, 71–72, 86
Parent-child relationship, dying children and, 40
Parents, of dying children, 29, 39, 40
Patient costs, hospice care and, 122, 135
Patterson, Bradford, 114–116, 120, 122, 127–128, 130–132
Pediatricians, parents of dying child and, 48
Personality factors
  individual response to death and, 41–42
  and people delaying treatment of cancer symptoms, 42

Pharmacies, in hospices, 61
Phenothiazine-compazine, 99
Physicians
  and admission to Hospice, Inc., 93
  avoidance of dying patients by, 50
  and dying children, 28–29
  fear of death and, 53
  of hospice patients, 64–65
  and management of bereavement, 45
  management of death by, 48–52
  volunteer, 77
Pilgrim Club, St. Christopher's, 78
Pleasure, dying patients and, 43, 71
Polypharmacy, 71–73
Population, age and sex distribution, 26
Poverty, cancer deaths and, 34
President's Cancer Panel, 140, 152–153
Privacy in hospice, 63, 74, 79, 103–104
Private sector, lag in response to hospice movement, 166

Prognosis, admission into Hospice Home Care Program and, 93
Public health movement, 23
Public Health Nurses, 119, 129
Punishment, disease viewed as, 43

Quality of life, hospices and, 73–74
Quint, Jeanne, 54

Race
  cancer incidence and, 30–34
  mortality rates and life expectancy by, 22, 23
Ravizza, Claire, 115, 117–120, 121, 122, 125, 127–132
Request for Proposals (RFP), from National Cancer Institute, hospices and, 159–163
Readmissions, at St. Christopher's, 80
Referral sources, to St. Christopher's, 81
Research
  on death fears, 41
  by National Cancer Institute, 140–141

[Research]
at St. Christopher's, 78
Revenues, at Hospice, Inc.,
109
Rosenblatt, Paul, 44
"Roving Clinic" at
Hospice, Inc., 95

Sachem Fund, 91, 93
St. Christopher's Hospice,
Sydenham, England,
65, 69–84
administrative structure
of, 69
admissions to, 70–71, 80,
81
age groups of patients
with malignant
diseases at, 82
cancer patients at, 81–82
clinical research at, 78
compared with Hospice,
Inc., 86
discharges from, 80
Domiciliary Service,
75–76
drug management at,
71–73
exclusion of pediatric
patients at, 119–120
families of patients at,
74–175
funding of, 76, 80

[St. Christopher's Hospice]
influence on Hospice,
Inc., 86–87, 95
length of stay for cancer
patients at, 82, 83
and National Cancer
Institute, 162
nursing care at, 73–74,
76
pain management at,
84
patient opinion of, 87
physical facilities at,
79–80
purpose of, 69–70
referral sources to, 81
staff selection and
training, 76–78
Study Center, 77–78
volunteers at, 77
St. Luke's Hospital, New
York City, 136–137
Saunders, Dr. Cicely, 63,
64, 65, 69, 71, 95
Schneidman, E. S., 45–46
Schoenberg, Bernard,
41–43, 44, 46, 49–50
Schowalter, John, 39–40
Schulz, Richard, 47
Senescu, Robert, 41–43, 44,
49–50
Separation anxiety, 39
Sex
cancer incidence and, 30

[Sex]
distribution of population
by, 26
mortality rates and life
expectancy by, 22, 23
Sexual relations, in hospice,
103–104
Social events, in hospice,
78–79
Staff
of Hospice, Inc., Home
Care Team, 95–97
lounges, 64, 105
meetings at St.
Christopher's, 76
proposed, for Strong
Hospice, 123
training at St.
Christopher's, 76
vacations for, 77
Strauss, Anselm, 47, 50–51
Strong Hospital Hospice,
proposal, 111–132, 133
administration, 124–125
budget estimates,
125–127
components of, 123–125
environment plan, 124
estimated use of, 118
exclusion of pediatric
patients from, 119–120
failure of, 127–132
feasibility study of,
116–120, 122–125

[Strong Hospital Hospice]
funding problems,
115–117, 125, 128–130
Home Care proposal, 124
interaction between
hospital and hospice,
123–124
recommendation on,
120–121
staff in, 123
support for, 115
Suicide rates, among
widowers, 44–45
Survivors, *See* Bereaved;
Family
Symptoms of dying
patients, 46, 69–70,
71–72, 83, 92, 98–99

Terminally ill, *See* Dying
children; Dying people
Terrill, Laura, 53
Third Party payments, 100,
108–109, 122, 130
Thompson, John, 14–15
Thorazine, 72
Toxicity, pain management
and, 73
Transitional spaces in
hospices, 64, 102

Van Amerigen Foundation,
91, 93, 129

Visitors, 61, 74, 94
Visiting Nurses, 16, 119, 129
"Visitors Day Off," 79
Volunteers in hospices, 65, 75, 77, 94, 97–98
Vomiting, 70, 98

Wald, Florence, 60–65, 86, 95–96
Walsh, Rose, 44
Ward patients, 54–55
Wessel, Dr. Morris, 86
"What is Hospice," 85
Widowers, 44–45

Widowhood, increase in, 25
Wiener, Jerry, 48

Yale-New Haven Hospital Hospice, Inc., and, 86, 87
rates per diem, compared with Hospice, Inc., 106
sources of reimbursement for patients dying at, 108–109

Zoning laws, hospices and, 106